Tackling the Kala-Azar Menace in Bihar

An Integrated Perspective

Tackling the Kala-Azar Menace in Bihar

An Integrated Perspective

Ganga Kumar
Ragini Mishra

PRABHAT PRAKASHAN
ISO 9001: 2008 Publishers

Published by
PRABHAT PRAKASHAN
4/19 Asaf Ali Road,
New Delhi-110 002 (INDIA)
Tele : +91-11-23289777
e-mail: prabhatbooks@gmail.com

ISBN 978-93-5186-522-3
TACKLING THE KALA-AZAR MENANCE IN BIHAR: An Integrative Perspective
by Ganga Kumar and Ragini Mishra

Edition
First, 2015

Price
₹ 300 (Rupees Three Hundred only)

Printed at
R-Tech Offset Printers, Delhi

Preface

Kala-Azar, i.e. *Visceral Leishmaniasis* (*VL*) is a menace to the state of Bihar, affecting a large chunk of population. One-third cases of Kala-Azar are reported from Bihar itself, as per report of WHO. Diagnosis and case detections are done by rk39. Miltefosine has been rolled out in 16 highly endemic districts of Bihar, whereas other districts have coverage of Amphotericin B. and Sodium Stibo Gluconate as the treatment drugs. Vector control is solely done by Indoor Residual Spray using DDT. In spite of our consistent efforts to tackle the menace of this vector-borne disease spanning over a decade, we have not been able to contain this disease in the State. What is more perplexing is the spreading of Kala-Azar foci to the never districts in the State of Bihar, which were previously completely free from the disease. Lack of community participation has been the major lacuna in successful implementation of the Kala-Azar Control Programme. There is an urgent need to reframe the strategies for Kala-Azar Control Programme shifting the special focus on community participation in targeting areas like case detection, case reporting and referral aspect as well as control through Indoor Residual Spray.

The Govt. of India has planned to eliminate Kala-Azar by 2015 with high level of political commitment, reducing annual *VL* incidence to 1/10,000 of the population. Although the incidence of the disease has decreased substantially in Bihar in last few years, yet a disconcerting feature has been its spread to newer foci (districts). Initially, the disease was endemic in 31 districts but recently it has spread to 33 districts. The case fatality rate has decreased over the years due to better case management but it is still substantial. The increase in reported number of cases has led to introduction of several incentives like free diets and compensation for loss of wages and involvement of ASHAs in the initiative to control Kala-Azar. There has been shifting of a large number of patients from private sector to public sector after introduction of oral drug (miltefosine) and intensive case search programmes. Besides these, other factors like complexity of the disease itself and human-induced factors like poverty, illiteracy and housing patterns also kept on contributing to the increase in the rate of transmission of the disease.

In addition to the Department of Health of the Govt. of Bihar, many developmental partners are also working in the State towards Kala-Azar elimination, but to our dismay each of them is working in isolation. What is needed here is a systematic and integrated approach towards tackling the menace of the disease.

The aim of this work is to draw the attention of readers as well as policymakers to secure integration of the isolated efforts towards elimination of Kala-Azar at one platform and to enforce newer evidence based strategies in the State.

Ganga Kumar
(Email: kumar.ganga@nic.in)
Ragini Mishra
(Email: ragini330@gmail.com)

Acknowledgements

There are quite a number of contributors to this work who deserve appreciations. We would like to express our gratitude to all of them. Our parents and family members deserve the commendable appreciations without whose sacrifice and inducements this exercise might not have been possible.

We are also grateful to the Department of Health and State Health Society, Govt. of Bihar for making us available the valuable data and information needed for analysis of the Kala-Azar situation as it exists in Bihar.

A lamp that does not glow cannot light another lamp!!

The opinion mentioned in this book is of personal opinion and it has nothing to do with Government activities.

Ganga Kumar
Ragini Mishra

Contents

1

Health Concerns – Historical and Constitutional Moorings

Health: An Introduction

The term 'health' is a very subjective one to the person concerned, and can mean different things to different people. There are people who consider themselves healthy if they do not have any disease or disability. Some people with only minor troubles may perceive themselves to be in poor health in case their concept of health involves a higher degree of well-being. Certain other people, who have any disease or disability, may, in spite of these problems, regard themselves healthy if they are able to manage their conditions of health in a manner without having any adverse impact on the way they live.

The main focus of the health-care sector has often been the presence or absence of sickness, disease, injury and disability in the population. However, this does not constitute the whole picture. According to the World Health Organization, health is "a state of complete physical, mental and social well-being and not merely the absence of disease or infirmity". This definition extends the notion of health to add to it a sense of positive well-being.

There are many dimensions to the concept of health – physical, mental and social. During times of difficulty, strengths in one particular area of health may be counted on to supplement weaknesses in other areas. For example, the physical ill health experienced by older people can be, at least partly, balanced by positive reserves of mental health, and/or a supportive social environment.

Present Health System: An Introduction

The existing state of public health in the country is so unsatisfactory that any attempt to improve the present position must necessarily involve drastic administrative measures. There is no denial of the fact that the morbidity and mortality levels in the country are still unacceptably high. These unsatisfactory health indices are, in turn, indications of the limited success of the public health system in meeting the curative requirements of the general population.

The objective of universal access to quality health-care, envisaged over half a century ago at the dawn of Independence, remains partially unrealized. Public health has effectively remained a low priority for the Indian states in terms of financing and political attention. Consequently, there has been a major and growing divergence between the policy rhetoric (Bhore Committee, Alma Ata Declaration) and actual implementation. This has contributed to the slow and inadequate improvement in the health-care facilities to the population at large.

The system of health-planning and decision-making has been highly centralized and top-down mechanism with minimal accountability. There has been little decentralized planning with least scope for genuine community initiatives. The failure for most State-supported community health worker schemes is one of the most striking outcomes of this sort of planning from above. The family planning programme has been the most dominant amongst various externally-imposed priorities. It attempts to reduce the poor as a substitute to poverty alleviation drawing scarce resources away from public health. It has distorted the whole public health system alienating it from the people themselves.

This phase has witnessed staggering health inequities, resurgence of communicable disease and emergence of an even more unregulated drug industry with spiralling drug prices adding to the current crisis in public health. Special health needs of women and children have become further side-lined or inadequately addressed, while vital concerns like violence as a public health issue still remains unrecognized and ineffectively addressed.

It seems to be an appropriate time to place the goal of universal access to health-care on the agenda of the goal for the millennium, and to rebuild a social consensus on the issue of public health.

While developing such initiatives, we can draw upon the legal and constitutional provisions for the Right to Health-care, the declared wish yet never fulfilled. The time has now come to secure such right to the people simultaneously redefining and expanding the horizon of health entitlements. It is high time to reclaim public health essentially as a universal goal under the framework of human rights.

Right to Health: An International Perspective

Right to health and availability of qualitative health services are issues which are relevant all over the world. Hence, these are basically the topics of debate at various international fora. In particular, the United Nations has been keen on adopting various resolutions to safeguard the interests of the health and well-being of the people at large.

The Universal Declaration of Human Rights states that: "Everyone has the right to a standard of living adequate for the health and well-being of himself and his family, including food, clothing, housing and medical care, and necessary social services, and the right to security in the event of unemployment, sickness, disability, widowhood, old age or other lack of livelihood in circumstances beyond his control."

The International Covenant on Economic, Social and Cultural Rights also says to the State parties that the present Convention recognise the right of everyone to the enjoyment of the highest attainable standard of physical and mental health. In addition to these, the Covenants on the Rights of the Child have all been framed to protect the health-care rights of women, children and other discriminated sections of the society.

Health and Health-care: A National Perspective

Health and health-care have been covered under the Constitution of India as well as in different legislations. The Constitution does not explicitly recognize right to health as a fundamental right, but implicitly recognises this by making provisions under the directive principle of the State policy. Different legislative enactments passed with regard to health and health-care deal more with the regulatory aspects rather than the right to health. It can be interpreted that these statutes recognize right to health in a given context in an indirect sense.

Constitutional Provisions for Right to Health-Care

Preamble

Preamble to the Constitution of India categorically directs the State to initiate measures aiming at improving the health of the people, which is inferable from the broader parameters of social and economic justice.

Fundamental Rights

Part III of the Constitution deals with various fundamental rights. A perusal of the same reveals the following fundamental rights that are relevant to the health and health-care of the people.

Equality Before Law: According to this fundamental right, the State shall not deny to any person equality before the law or equal protection of the law within the territory of India.

Protection of Life and Personal Liberty: According to this fundamental right, no person shall be deprived of his life or personal liberty except according to the procedure established by law.

Directive Principles of State Policy

Essential premise of the principles enshrined in Part IV of our Constitution is to provide direction to the central and various State Governments to undertake and initiate required measures in the interests of the community. With regard to health and health-care, the following principles have direct bearing on which the States must strive to secure.

- That the health and strength of workers, men and women, and the tender age of children are not abused and that citizens are not forced by economic necessity to enter vocations unsuited to their age or strength;
- That children are given opportunities and facilities to develop in a healthy manner and in conditions of freedom and dignity and that childhood and youth are protected against exploitation and against moral and material abandment.
- *Right to Work, to Education and to Public Assistance in Certain Cases:* The State shall, within the limits of its economic capacity and development, make effective provision for securing

the right to work, to education and to public assistance in cases of unemployment, old age, sickness and disablement, and in other cases of undeserved want.

- *Provision for Just and Humane Conditions of Work and Maternity Relief:* The State shall make provision for securing just and humane conditions of work and for maternity relief.
- *Living Wages for Workers:* The state shall endeavour to secure, by suitable legislation or economic organisation or in any other way, to all workers, agricultural, industrial or otherwise, work, a living wage, conditions of work ensuring a decent standard of life and full enjoyment of leisure and social and cultural opportunities and, in particular, the State shall endeavour to promote cottage industries on an individual or co-operative basis in rural areas.
- *Duty of the State to Raise the Level of Nutrition and the Standard of Living and to Improve Public health:* The State shall regard the raising of the level of nutrition and standard of living of its people and the improvement of public health as among its primary duties, and in particular, the State shall endeavour to bring about prohibition of the consumption except for medicinial purposes of intoxicating drinks and of drugs which are injurious to health.

Fundamental Duties

Fundamental duties incorporated under Article 51A envisages some pertinent principles to be followed by every citizen of India, which are relevant for health concerns and reads as under:

- To protect and improve the natural environment including forests, lakes, rivers and wild life, and to have compassion for living creatures;

- To develop the scientific temper, humanism and the spirit of inquiry and reform;
- To strive towards excellence in all spheres of individual and collective activity so that the nation constantly rises to higher levels of endeavour and achievement.

□

2

Menace of Kala-Azar: Indian Scenario

Kala-Azar or *Visceral Leishmaniasis* is a complex disease caused by a protozoan, Leishmania and transmitted by the vector *Phlebotomus argentipes*, commonly known as sandfly. In India, the endemic belt includes Meghalaya, Assam (Brahmaputra Valley), Bihar, West Bengal, Eastern Uttar Pradesh, Coastal Andhra Pradesh and Tamil Nadu.

Kala-Azar was first reported in Jessore district of West Bengal in the year 1824-25, and was known as 'Jwar-vikar' at that time. Kala-Azar cases were recorded in different districts of West Bengal since 1931 (Napier, 1931). In Assam, the disease was first found in the year 1869 with sporadic occurrence in Garo Hills followed by a regular epidemic at an interval of 15 years till 1944. In Bihar, it was first recorded as "Kala-dukh" in Purnea district in 1882 (Bora, 1999). The notable epidemics were observed in 1891, 1917 and 1933. The endemicity of the disease continued till sixties with a marked decline thereafter. An epidemic periodicity of every 20 years has been postulated for kala-azar. Gravity of the situation was such that hardly any control mechanism was available against the vector, and obviously no drugs were there to cure the patients.

Population growth and economic development were considered to be an important indicator for the spread of this disease. A painstaking study done by Young revealed that when the population growth increased by 15-20% per decade, there was high kala-azar-mortality rate, but in another case in Assam, a decline in Kala-Azar cases was observed. It was found to primarily affect the children and young adults that sapped the vitality of the population.

A very famous Hindi novel named 'Maila Aanchal' written by great regional novelist Faneeshwar Nath 'Renu' reflects the incidence and fears of Kala-Azar, as the hero of the novel Dr. Prashant was very much keen on the research activities on the Kala-Azar in the area of Purnea district in North Bihar. Kala-Azar had been so endemic in Bihar, Bengal province and Assam that the British Government had formed a 'Kala-Azar Commission' in the mid-twenty of the twentieth century. The Commission first time proved that this disease was not spread by direct infection or food and water contamination but due to the biting of female sand-flies of a particular species named *Phlebotomus argentipes*. This commission also proved that unicellular parasites named *Leishmania donovani* (named after Leishman and Donovan) remains the sole cause of *Visceral Leishmaniasis* in India and it is spread by the vector sandflies, *P. argentipes*.

As a consequence of withdrawal of DDT spray under National Malaria Eradication Programme (NMEP) from Kala-Azar endemic areas in 1963-64, the disease resurgence occurred in late seventies because of slow build-up of vector population. Currently, the disease has been found to be endemic only in Bihar, West Bengal and eastern part of Uttar Pradesh adjoining Bihar (Bora, 1998; Chandra, 1995 and Marwaha, 1991). The disease occurs in sporadic, endemic and epidemic forms in different geographical regions of these States. Kala-Azar cases started being reported from many hospitals in North Bihar districts from 1974 onwards only. However, by 1977, several districts of Bihar started reporting fresh cases and then onwards the problem became a regular phenomenon in the entire northern districts and some of the districts situated south of river Ganges in Bihar. The State witnessed two major epidemic outbreaks of Kala-Azar in the year 1978 and 1992. The first person to consider the possible association of the genus *Phlebotomus* with the transmission of Kala-Azar was Mackie, who once remarked, "The only insect which has given any return for work put into it is the sandfly, and I am of the opinion that the relation of this insect to the disease would repay further investigation."

The association of *Phlebotomus argentipes* and Kala-Azar was also pointed out by Shortt and Swaminath. There has been little doubt that Mackie in 1914 when working on Kala-Azar in Assam actually dissected *P. argentipes* although he was not aware of its identity at that time.

In 1922, Swaminath of the Kala-Azar enquiry team of the Indian Research Fund Association (IRFA) in Assam under the direction of Major H.E. Shortt IMS, again dissected *P. argentipes*, but without positive identification. In 1922, Major JAS Inton VC, I.M.S. in a private communication to Lt. Colonel R. Knowles IMS pointed out that the known distribution of *P. argentipes* in India corresponds closely with that of Kala-Azar.

The Kala-Azar Commission was sanctioned by Govt. of India in April 1924. The officers appointed included Lieut. Col. S.R. Cristopher CIE, OBM, IMS (Director), Major H.E. Shortt, IMS Protozoologist and Mr. P.J. Barraud, Entomologist. Kala-Azar Enquiry Committee consisted of Major R. Knowles, Dr. L.E. Napier and Military Assistant Surgeon, R.O.A. Smith. The Enquiry Committee was constituted primarily to study *Culicoides* and *Phlabotomus,* and that work actually commenced in Assam. Though a few insects like bed-bug and blood sucking individuals of the genus *Triatoma* were suspected to transmit Kala-Azar on account of their presence in Kala-Azar endemic areas in India, yet negative results were obtained after feeding on Kala-Azar patients by Donovan (1913) and Cornwal (1916). With regard to mosquitoes, Mackie examined 266 Culex species and 18 Anopheles fed on Kala-Azar patients but negative results were obtained.

Certain non-blood sucking insects such as the house fly, and cockroach were suggested as mechanical carriers or hosts, but there appears to be nothing in support of such views. Among the worms, leech and two ankylostomes were also suspected to be the possible carriers but again negative results were found. In general, therefore, the attempt to implicate any arthropod or other blood sucking host up to the time of the commission's commencing work was found to be negative. Mackie in his paper "Insects and Kala-Azar" aptly remarked about the suspicion of insect vectors in transmission of Kala-Azar.

Some scientists have hypothesized various ways by which the infection of Kala-Azar may occur. These ways were speculated to include direct contagious spread or transmission via intestinal discharges or by ingestion but again only negative results were found. On account of the peculiar topographical distribution of Kala-Azar in India, Short at first suggested that sandfly appears to be the insect vector in 1922 and in the same year Napier found a close correspondence between the distribution of *P. argentipes* and the number of Kala-Azar cases and noted that this species of sandfly feeds solely on man.

From November 1923 to April 1924, some *Phlebotomine* flies were dissected and for the first time, some of the flies dissected were definitely identified as *P. argentipes*. In February 1924, Shortt gave probably the first published record of *P. argentipes* in Assam in a paper read before the Assam branch of the British Medical Association. In this paper, the suspected transmitters of

Kala-Azar were classified into groups as 'probable' and 'possible', placing the genus *Phlabotomus* under the former group. This paper was read previous to the actual dissection of the first *P. argentipes* on 17 March 1924 and the presences of mammalian blood in these vectors were observed. In December 1924, connection between *Phlebotomus* and Kala-Azar was confirmed. Knowles, Napier and Smith published a note entitled "On a herpetomonas found in the gut of the sandfly *P. argentipes* fed on Kala-Azar patients". These workers showed that the parasites in the peripheral blood of a Kala-Azar patient in the form of Leishman-Donovan bodies become converted into flagellate forms in the gut of laboratory bred *P. argentipes*. This important discovery immediately brought the focus on the genus *Phlabotomus* and ending the discursive efforts on a variety of suspected insects as carriers for the disease of Kala-Azar. This discovery was quickly confirmed by the Kala-Azar Commission.

In March 1925, Christopher, Shortt and Barraud gave the first description of the flagellates encountered in the infected flies and of their location in the gut of the insect. They also described for the first time the invasion of the pharynx of the flies by the flagellates. In April 1925, the same workers used a series of controls with laboratory-bred flies and proved that the flagellates seen in the *P. argentipes* after feeding on Kala-Azar cases were *Leishmania donovani* in reality. In July 1925, P.J. Barraud FES of the Kala-Azar Commission made a sandfly survey of Madras city and found four species of *Phlabotomus*. Up to this time, the great difficulty experienced in all experiments to prove the transmission of Kala-Azar by the bite of the sandfly was laid in the fact that the fed flies almost invariably died by the fifth day after initial feed and before the second feed could be taken. The cause of the death was found to be invariably due to the failure of the fly to oviposit, without which the act of second blood meal could not become possible.

In September 1925, the commission overcame this difficulty by the discovery of a technique which enabled the flies to oviposit and take many successive meals with oviposition occurring between each two meals. This technique opened up the way to an extensive series of transmission experiments by the Kala-Azar Commission and other workers. In November 1925, as a direct result of the application of this technique Shortt, Barraud and Craighead discovered massive infections of the pharynx and the buccal cavity in *P. argentipes* that had received two or three blood meals. By December 1925, the same workers elucidated for the first time the complete life history of *L. donovani* in *P. argentipes*, and this work was subsequently published in April 1926. In February 1926, the Kala-Azar Memoir (Memoir-4) was published. Besides the work already alluded to the memoir, it contained a description of the anatomy of the head of the *P. argentipes* which was published under three names. Among the included papers, one was written by Napier and Smith on the bionomics of *P. argentipes* with special reference to the conditions in Calcutta. Napier published a paper entitled "Epidemiological Consideration of the Transmission of Kala-Azar." In this paper, twenty one conditions were laid down as favourable for the hypothetical transmission of Kala-Azar but many of these did not even stand the test of universal application even in India alone.

In May 1926, a technique was elaborated by the Kala-Azar Commission for breeding of *P. argentipes* throughout the year on a large scale by artificial rearing methods. In June 1926, Shortt, Barrud and Craighead described the occurrence of a massive infection of the buccal cavity of *P. argentipes* with *L. donovani* in which the most anteriorly placed flagellates protruded from the mouth part of the fly. It was found that such a fly in attempting to feed transferred some of its flagellates to the wounds. In July 1926, the commission caught the first specimen of *P. argentipes* in nature that showed infection with *L. donovani*. In September 1926, Shortt, Barrud and Craighead showed that the forms of *L. donovani* found in *P. argentipes* were infective to mice when inoculated intraperitoneal. At the same time, a study was completed regarding Row's body relationship to the production of the infection. In September 1926, experiments related to this topic were started with human volunteers but in October 1927 first series of transmission experiments with human volunteers were completed. In January 1928, it was demonstrated for the first time that the parasites *L. donovani* remained present in the nodules of dermal leishmaniasis patients, similar to those taken from the peripheral circulation of Kala-Azar cases.

In April 1928, Chinese hamsters (*Cricetulus griseus*) were found to be infected for the first time by the oral and the conjunctival routes and in the same year, the presence of *P. argentipes* infected with *L. donovani* was found in nature. In May 1929, numerous natural breeding places of *P. argentipes* were discovered. At the same time, it was demonstrated that the infection of healthy hamsters became possible if they were kept along with the infected hamsters and a group of *P. argentipes*. In June 1931, a hamster was found to be infected with Kala-Azar when it was fed by *P. argentipes* infected with *L. donovani*.

It was finally proved at the end of the Kala-Azar Commission in 1934 that for the spread of Kala-Azar in human being there occurs no other way of transmission than that of the bite of *P. argentipes*. After the publication of the report of Kala-Azar Commission, many workers in the field traced the relation of *Leishmania donovani* with *P. argentipes*. With further improvement of techniques, the methods being followed improved and laboratory based rearing of sandflies was also successfully done.

The final confirmations of the transmission of Kala-Azar by *P. argentipes* were shown by Swaminath C.S., Shortt H.E. and Anderson, L.A.P. in 1942. After confirmation of interrelation of sandfly and Kala-Azar, many works were done on the bionomics of sandflies. Bionomic studies established the presence of 42 species of sandflies in India. In the area of bionomics of sandflies, landmark works have been done by Lewis (1978) and Sanyal (1979).

Before the introduction of specific treatment in 1922, the mortality due to Kala-Azar was found to vary from 90-95%. Pentavalent antimony compounds which was first introduced by U.N. Brahmchari as urea stibamine, still remained the sheet anchor of treatment against Kala-Azar. The use of statistics in the field of vector biology research was formulated by Udney and Kandall in 1958 in London and reformed by Martin Blend.

The statistical analysis helped much in the epidemiological study of Kala-Azar. In 1979, Sanyal, R.K., Alam, S.N., Kaul, S.M. and Wattal, B.L. worked on the epidemiology of Kala-Azar in Bihar. In 1977, the technique was reformed by Killck-Kendric, Leaney, A.J. and Reddy, P.D. The statistical technique was further modified for *Phlebotomus* species by Modi, G.B. and Tesh, R.B. in 1983.

Just after independence, the Health Ministry of the Govt. of India, focussed mainly on the Malaria Programme and initiated the National Malaria Control Programme in 1953. This programme was reformed in 1958, but with little focus on Kala-Azar. In 1977, Kala-Azar was made a part of Malaria Eradication Plan of the Union Government. In 1990-91, the Central Government initiated the Kala-Azar Control Programme for the first time.

In the National Health Policy, 2002, it was declared that this disease would be eradicated completely by the end of the next eight years. In the mid-1950s, a gradual decline of Kala-Azar cases was observed to a point of almost total disappearance within a decade. The causes of disappearance of Kala-Azar were critically reviewed. However, effective treatment of the cases, increase in solid immunity, and consequent inter-epidemic lull and also the impact of DDT sprays under the National Malaria Eradication Programme were the reasons for the decline Kala-Azar cases.

Menace of Kala-Azar in Bihar

However, the disease after remaining dormant for sometimes, again assumed epidemic proportions in north Bihar by 1975-76 and the condition became worst in 1977 when major Kala-Azar outbreak occurred. In Bihar initially out of 38 districts, 31 districts were endemic for Kala-Azar but recent trend shows that the foci of the Kala-Azar has expanded to 33 districts which is the cause of concern.

In recent successive two years of 2012 and 2013, Kala-Azar cases show remarkable decline. This may partly be attributed to better case management and camp-based search of cases. However, this has to be closely monitored as the prevalence is still high considering the time period of Kala-Azar elimination by 2015 in the State.

□

3

Vector and its Life Cycle

Phlebotomus argentipes is a small, dark brown, hairy insect of about the length of 2.5 mm from the tip of mouth parts to the last abdominal segment. It belongs to the sub-family *Phlebotominae* which comprises more than 600 species. Of about 50 species of sandflies present in India, the subfamily *Phlebotominae* comprises six genera, viz. *Phlebotomus*, *Sergentomiya*, *Brumptomiya*, *Luyzomiya*, *Warileya* and *Parvideus*. Out of these, only two genera viz., *Phlebotomus* and *Sergentomiya* have been recorded from the Indian subcontinent. About 600 species of sandflies have been reported from various parts of the world, out of which about 46 species have been recorded from India (*Phlebotomus*-11, *Sergentomiya*-35).

In Bihar, as many as 31 species of sandflies have been found but generally three species remain significant. These three species include *Phlebotomus argentipes*, *Phlebotomus papatasi* and *Sergentomyia babu*. *P. argentipes* is the only species that transmits Kala-Azar to man.

P. argentipes has a very wide distribution range stretching from Iran to Indonesia. But the core area of its distribution range lies in the eastern and south eastern India. It is because of availability of the alluvial soil, high humidity, relatively equable temperatures and abundance of cattle population, it is able to build up enormous population densities, and to transmit Kala-Azar.

Sandfly is 1/3rd the size of the mosquito and has high tendency to breed in warm and moist places and its prevalence in Bihar is attributed to the environmental factors. The colours of sandflies vary species-wise. The colour of *P. argentipes* is light brown, the colour of P. *papatasi* is pale yellowish and that of *Sergentomyia sp.* is brown. All the species of the sandflies have dense hairy projections all over the body segments. Sandflies have one pair of compound eyes, respectively very long legs and almost erected wings. The wings of the sandflies are also covered by hairs.

Life Cycle of Sandflies

The life cycle of sandflies resembles that of mosquitoes in the basic pattern. It comprises four stages, i.e. the eggs, larval stage, the non-feeding pupal stage and the adult stage. However, sand flies including the vector *P. argentipes* breed in moist soil unlike mosquitoes which breed in water. Having originated from aquatic larvae of *Psychodidae* in the evolutionary process, the larvae of *Phlebotomine* sand flies become adapted to live in moist soil. The larvae therefore cannot exist without water in fluid form.

The larvae, particularly the younger instar, have been observed to absorb water with their food and through the skin. Confirming to these requirements, the female sandflies have been found to lay eggs in moist places at humidity levels approaching hundred percent. Such conditions are present in the forest soil, burrows, leaf litter and around tree bases. In arid conditions or biotopes, the sandflies seek micro-habitats meeting the breeding requirements and this accounts for association of large population of sand flies to termite hills and in gerbil burrows, particularly lining the river banks or pond banks.

Therefore, the distribution becomes uneven largely due to the effect of soil chemistry and moisture. The larvae after hatching out from the eggs penetrate some inches below the surface of the substrate. The larva, feed on decaying organic matters.

The larval stage further comprises its four sub-stages, which lead to progressive growth and last for about 10 days. The larval stage is followed by the non-feeding pupal stage which lasts about 7-10 days under optimum conditions. The larvae are very small with body covered with numerous chaetae which glue substrate particles and mask them. That is the reason only older larvae and pupae can be found in soil samples after most careful searches. No eggs or younger larvae of sandflies have ever been found in nature. Eggs and larvae of *P. argentipes* can withstand immersion in water for considerable time. First stage larvae can survive immersion for five days, and larvae of the 4th stage for 14 days.

These findings possibly explain the survival of larvae in the soil during the heavy monsoon rains when their breeding places may be flooded. Breeding places of *P. argentipes* are found within a radius of about 20 yards of a dwelling house, in dark, humid soil protected from sunlight. In the cattle sheds, the favourite breeding place is the floor underneath the earthenware trough. *P. argentipes* does not breed in rodent burrows, outside or in the dwellings. After emergence, the adults feed and mate within about 24-48 hours. The males often form swarms on buffalos seeking mating females. Female sandflies require a blood meal for egg development and maintenance of water balance. They also imbibe plant juices, a fact of considerable epidemiological importance as the capacity of *Phlebotomus argentipes* to transmit *L. donovani* is enhanced by feeding plant juices. Only the female sandflies are haematophagous, i.e. take a blood meal. *Phlebotomus argentipes* prefers cattle blood to human. But during the transmission season from June to October, when there is a tremendous build-up of *P. argentipes* densities, there is a spill over of population into human dwellings, enhancing man-vector contact. During feeding, saliva is introduced into the host, one component of which is a peptide considered to be one of the most potent vasodilators ever discovered. Sandfly saliva enhances the growth of *Leishmania* in the host.

In the Assam State, and adjoining plains of the north-eastern India, *P. argentipes*, has apparently been eliminated by continuous anti-malaria spraying. In these states, no indigenous Kala-Azar has been reported since the 1950s except in year 2005 when one case was reported from the state of Assam. In addition to blood, sandflies also ingest cells lying in the dermis outside the blood circulation and thus infected macrophages may be picked up. Life cycle of sandfly is completed in the moist soil unlike mosquito which breeds in water. Because of this, the anti-larval insecticides or other chemical and biological control methods used in mosquito control cannot be applied to sandfly.

Moreover, due to high fertile land in Bihar and flooding, and especially water-logging for a long period due to poor drainage system constitutes the whole land favourable for the breeding of the sandfly. Feeding on the plant juices during the pre-transmission period is again favourable due to the greeneries found in Bihar.

Systematic position of Sandflies in India

Phylum—*Arthropoda*
Class—*Insecta*
Sub-class—*Pterygota*
Order—*Diptera*
Sub-order—*Orthorrapha*
Group—*Nematocera*
Family—*Psychodidae*
Sub-family—*Phlebotominae*
Genus—*Phlebotomus/Sergentomyia/Papatasi*.

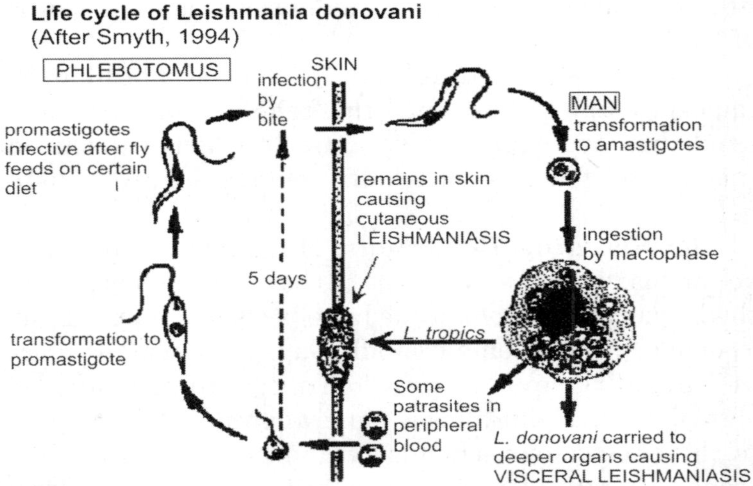

Fig. 1. Life Cycle of *Leishmania donovani* is completed in two host—1. Sandflies. and 2. Man

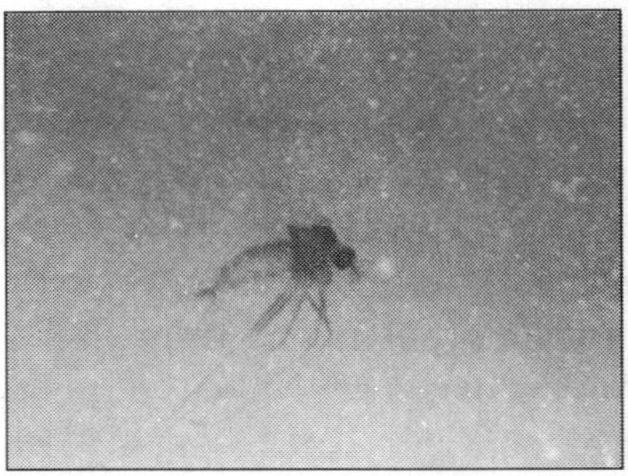

Fig. 2. Male *P. argentipes*

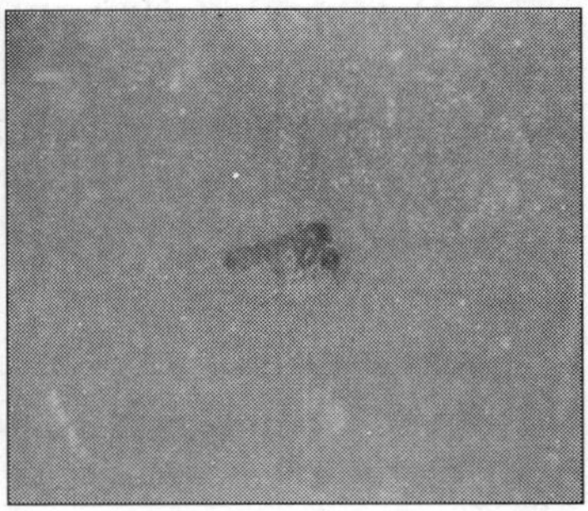

Fig. 3. Female *P. argentipes*

Bionomics of Sandflies

For the prevention of *Visceral Leishmaniasis*, the control of its vectors in Sandflies is mandatory. This target can only be attained when the bionomics of this vector is properly known. Study of each and every stage of sand-flies helps understanding the effects of environmental and climatic factors on them. This interrelationship would help entomologists/public health experts/health department for successful control of this vector.

All types of studies on sand flies would prove imperfect unless and until the behavioural patterns of sand flies are explored fully. Certain generalized and interesting features of sandfly bionomics are enlisted below:

(i) *Breeding Behaviour*: Having originated from aquatic larvae of *Psychodidae* in the evolutionary process, the larvae of *Phlebotominae* have become adapted to live in moist soil. The female sandfly lays eggs in moist places at humidity levels approaching hundred percent. Distribution of sandflies is generally uneven largely due to the effect of soil chemistry and moisture. Immature stages are often found in loose soil in cracks and closely packed earth, collected near the dwelling houses or cattle sheds.

(ii) *Feeding Behaviour*: The adult sandflies prefer glucose and fructose and few types of amino-acids as their food. Males strictly depend on plant juices. During routine sandfly collection, and general field survey, it has been found that the sandflies prefer some plants more than others. Those plants which are avoided and disliked by the sandflies can be useful as the repellent against them. In general, females of the *Phlebotomus argentipes* depend upon the mammals for their blood meal (Kaul et al., 1979).

(iii) *Resting Behaviour*: Sandflies have a wide range of resting habits which may vary from species to species. They generally rest in a shelter having diffused light, high relative humidity ranging from 80-85% and temperature ranging from 25-30°C. *P. argentipes* is an endophilic species. In cattle sheds, they rest in cracks and crevices of mud plastered floors and walls. In human dwellings also, they rest in cracks and crevices of brick walls near the ground surface where coolness and dampness prevail. During resting, they place their antennae downward making an acute angle with respect to the surface. It has been found that the hind legs of sand-flies remain in tensile condition even when they rest and as soon as it is disturbed it first hops and then flies.

(iv) ***Light and Dispersal Habits*****:** Sandflies are incapable of flying long distances and generally move by their characteristic hopping movements. It has been found that the sandfly first lowers its abdomen and the very long hind legs are compressed like a spring. Perhaps, the flight physiology of the sandfly shows that it costs too much of its stored energy and so the sandflies mainly disperse by its hopping movements and fly only rarely when flight remains the only option of dispersal.

(v) ***Mating Behaviour*****:** Role of sounds produced by both sexes of sandflies and pheromones produced by female sandflies is very much important in the courtship behaviour of the sandflies. Female sandflies secrete some special pheromones and these also make some special noise to attract the male individuals. The females are engaged in sucking blood meal from their mammalian host and have never been found to take part in any kind of courtship acts except secretion of pheromones and special noise. The courtship actions are performed actively by the male sandflies mainly. After one or two days of the mating, females require one or two blood meal again to mature the eggs and after the optimum cycles of the blood meals, the female engage in search of suitable cracks and places where they can lay eggs. The abdominal colour of the gravid female turn brownish and the last segment of the gravid females become rounded and swollen. After two or three days, the female lay eggs inside the safe places with the optimum environmental conditions and on an average in ninety-two percent of cases it has been found that female sandflies die out after the successful oviposition.

(vi) ***Seasonal Dynamics*****:** High densities of *P. argentipes* seem to be pre-requisite for Kala-Azar transmission. Transmission season of Kala-Azar in India is coincidental with the season of the highest *P. argentipes* densities, which is from June to October. In the north-east India, *P. argentipes* vanishes during the cold months of December and January and reappears in small numbers in March. The numbers shoot up dramatically after the onset of monsoon and remain high till the end of October.

A study on the monthly vector density study was carried out by the State Surveillance Unit, Bihar. Two sentinel sites were fixed in 2012 for collection where several houses and other dwellings were searched for the presence of sandflies. One place was Village Tope which lies in PHC Daniyawan of district Patna, while other is Village Malpur Singhara, which lies in PHC Mahua of District Vaishali. Village Tope was selected as 'Control village', as it was non-endemic for Kala-Azar since past few years, whereas Village Singhara was used as 'Case Village', as it was endemic for Kala-Azar.

Collections were done using hand aspirator and torch light in cattle sheds, human dwellings and mixed dwellings in early morning and at the dusk hours. Maximum collections were done from mixed dwellings>cattle sheds>human dwellings. In human dwellings three categories of houses were searched, viz. Thatched (bamboo sheds), *Kutcha* (brick and mud plaster or mud and soil) and *Pucca* (concrete). House index of sandflies were more in Thatched houses>*Kutcha* houses>*Pucca* houses.

A remarkable feature was noticed during the survey. No Kala-Azar cases were reported from Village Tope, Patna since last three years as a result of which the village was not covered under the spray micro plan. As a result of discontinuation of spray activities, vector population was found to resurge in village Tope due to which vector density in that village was found to be more than village

Singhara in Vaishali District, an area otherwise endemic for Kala-Azar.

The study of monthly vector density was correlated with monthly reported cases of vector-borne diseases in the State and found to be useful in generating early warning Signals (EWS) of impending vector-borne outbreaks in the State. Health alerts were issued to districts in case increase in vector density and numbers of cases were noticed. Vector density survey was also carried after spray activities in Vaishali District.

The results showed that the spray activities reduced vector density and if it is carried out regularly, the same would help in containing vector population in the spray areas. The study also led to conclusion that complete rather than focal spray would be more useful if we have to contain the vectors. The study also throws light on carrying the monthly vector density surveys in each district on a regular basis for which involvement of Vector Borne Disease Consultants, Epidemiologists, Kala-Azar Technical Supervisor and other surveillance workers would prove to be useful. This would further help in containing the burden of vector-borne diseases in the State.

Month, wise vector density graph based on monthly survey is represented as under:

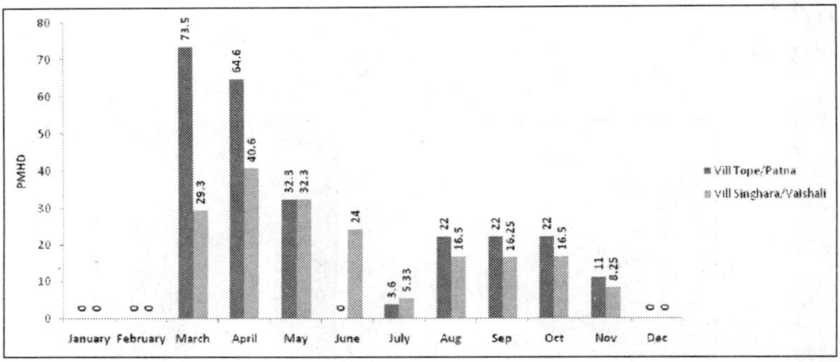

Fig. 4. Monthwise PMHD of female sandflies in Vill tope, Patna & Vill Singhara, vaishali in 2012

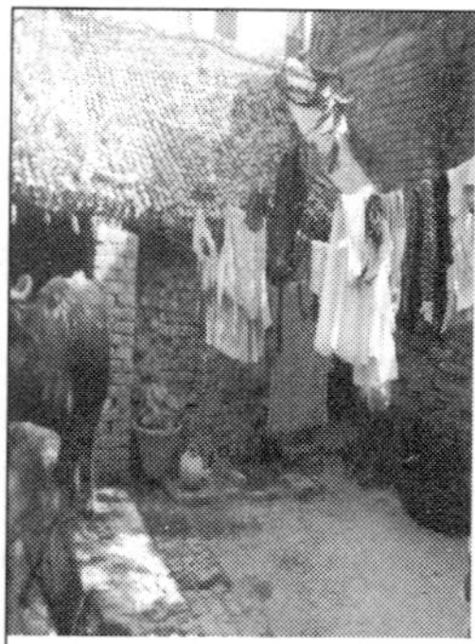

Mixed Dwellings, Vill: Tope, PHC Daniyawan, Patna

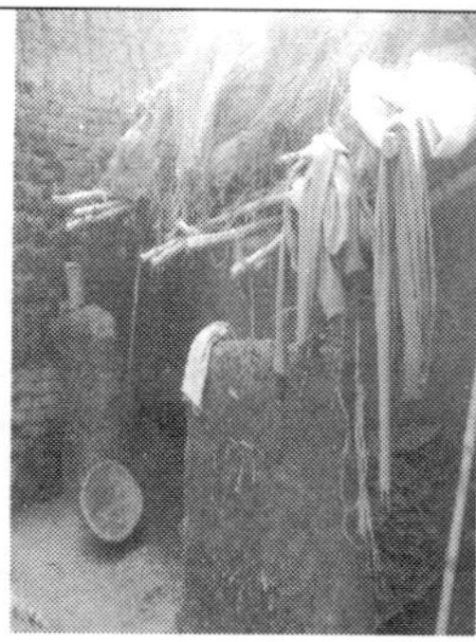

Cow dung plastered houses, Vill: Malpur Singhara, Vaishali

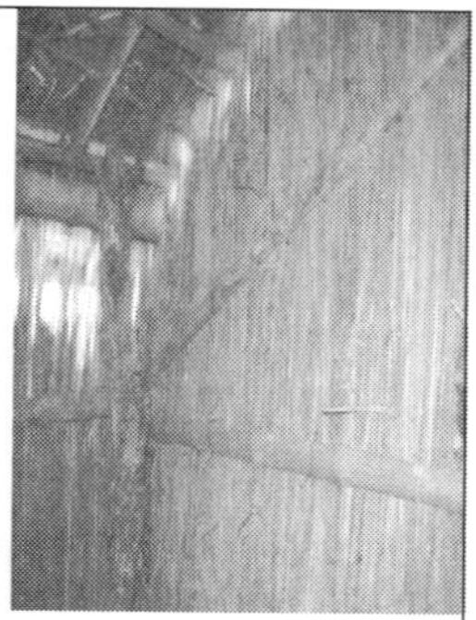

Thatched bamboo huts, Vill: Malpur Singhara, Vaishali

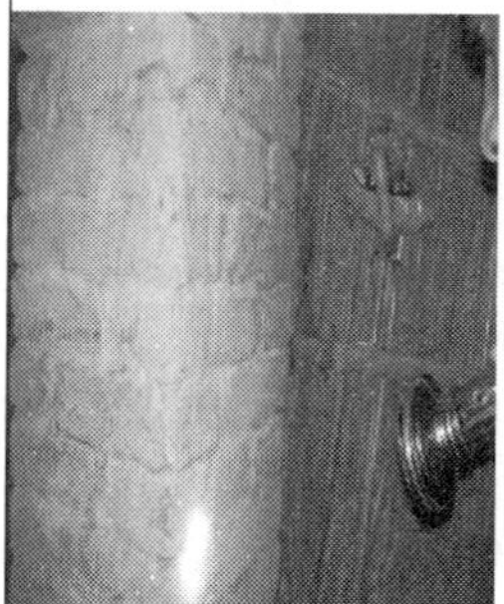

Thatched houses with brick walls, Vill: Tope, Patna

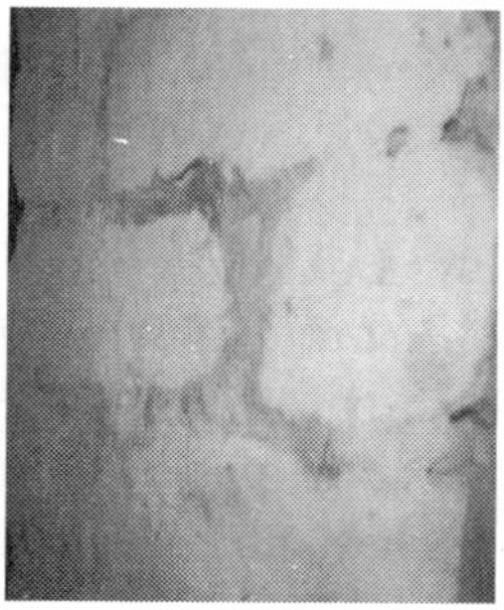

Cracks in brick walls where sandflies were found, Vill: Malpur Singhara, Vaishali

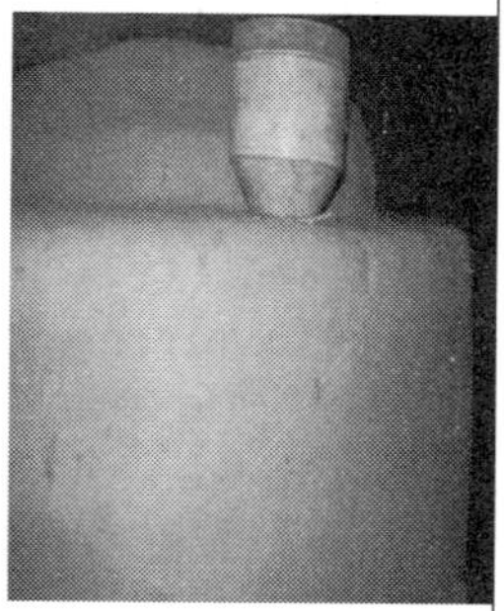

Earthen mounds for cereal storage, sandflies found near its base, Vill: Tope, Patna

Fig. 5. Different types of habitats from where sandflies were caught(Vill: Tope, Patna &Vill:Singhara,Vaishali)

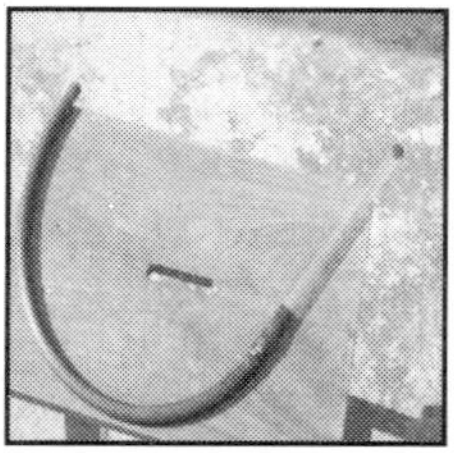

Fig. 6. Suction Tube for Catching Sandflies

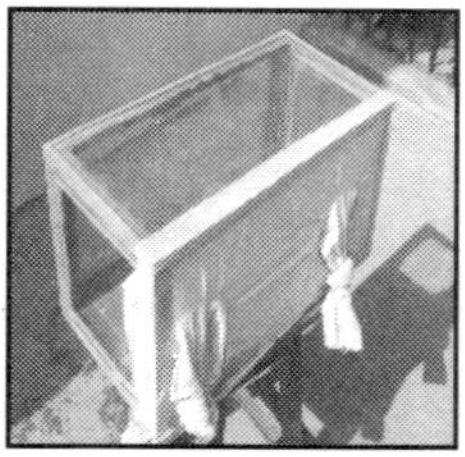

Fig. 7. Rearing Cage For Sandflies

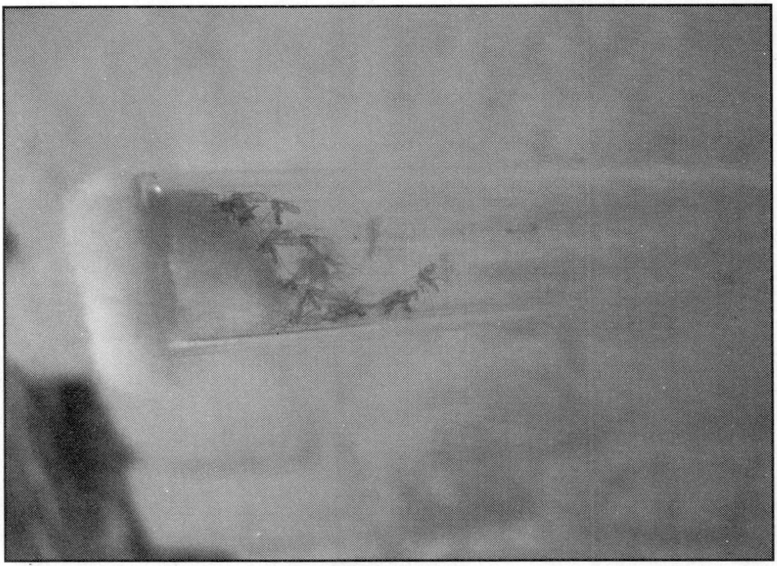

Fig 8: Sandflies collected in the field

□

4

Parasite and its Life Cycle

Leishmania donovani is an intracellular parasitic protozoan belonging to the genus *Leishmania* which causes the disease leishmaniasis. It is a human blood parasite responsible for *Visceral leishmaniasis* or kala-azar, the most severe form of leishmaniasis. It infects the mononuclear phagocyte system including spleen, liver and bone marrow. Infection is transmitted by species of sandfly belonging to the genus *Phlebotomus* in Old World and *Lutzomyia* in New World. Therefore, the parasite is prevalent throughout tropical and temperate regions including Africa (mostly in Sudan), China, India, Nepal, southern Europe, Russia and South America. It is responsible for thousands of deaths every year and has spread to 88 countries with 350 million people at constant risk of infection and occurrence of 0.5 million new cases in a year.

L. donovani was independently discovered in Madras, India, in 1903 by two British medical officers William Boog Leishman and Charles Donovan. However, the correct taxonomy was provided by Ronald Ross. The parasite requires two different hosts for a complete life cycle, humans as the definitive host and sandflies as the intermediate host. In some parts of the world, other mammals, especially canines, act as reservoir hosts. In human cell, they exist as small, spherical and unflagellated amastigote form; while they are elongated with flagellum as promastigote form in sandflies. Unlike other parasitic protists they are unable to directly penetrate the host cell, and are dependent upon phagocytosis.

Classification

Eukaryota; Euglenozoa; Kinetoplastida; Trypanosomatidae; Leishmania; Leishmania donovani.

Leishmaniasis is caused by a protozoa parasite from over 20 *Leishmania* species and is transmitted to humans by the bite of infected female phlebotomine sandflies. There are three main forms of the disease:

- *Visceral leishmaniasis* (*VL* also known as kala-azar) is fatal if left untreated. It is characterized by irregular bouts of fever, weight loss, enlargement of the spleen & liver and anaemia. It is highly endemic in the Indian subcontinent and in East Africa. An estimated 200000 to 400000 new cases of *VL* occur worldwide each year. Over 90% of new cases occur in six countries: Bangladesh, Brazil, Ethiopia, India, South Sudan, and Sudan.
- *Cutaneous Leishmaniasis* (*CL*) is the most common form of *leishmaniasis* and causes ulcers on exposed parts of the body, leaving life long scars and serious disability. About 95% of *CL* cases occur in the American, the Mediterranean basin, and the Middle East and Central Asia. Over two-third of *CL* new cases occur in six countries: Afghanistan, Algeria, Brazil, Colombia, Islamic Republic of Iran and the Syrian Arab Republic. An estimated 0.7 million to 1.3 million new cases occur worldwide annually.
- *Mucocutaneous leishmaniasis* leads to partial or total destruction of mucous membranes of the nose, mouth and throat. Almost 90% of *Mucocutaneous*

leishmaniasis cases occur in the Plurinational State of Bolivia, Brazil and Peru.

Life Cycle

Infection occurs when infected sandfly regurgitates infective promastigotes into the blood while feeding. The promastigotes are phagocytised by macrophages and transformed into amastigotes which multiply by binary fission in the macrophages. The life cycle is continued when a sandfly feeds on an infected person and ingests the amastigotes in the macrophages.

Symptoms/Pathology

Infection with *Leishmania* species can result in three main types of disease depending on the species' geographic region and host immune response. *Leishmania donovani* produces *Visceral leishmaniasis* (Kala-Azar). Symptoms include fever (often two fever spikes per day), enlargement of the spleen and liver, weakness, and progressive emaciation. The disease is often fatal without treatment but survivors often develop immunity. *Leishmania Tropica* and *L. mexicana* produce *Cutaneous leishmaniasis* which is characterized by skin lesions (oriental sore). Infected *Macrophages* containing amastigotes are found primarily at the site of infection around the sores. The sores are characterized by an elevated rim encircling the lesion. The sores generally heal by themselves within a year, but secondary bacterial infections are possible in open sores. *Leishmania braziliensis* produces *Mucocutaneous leishmaniasis*, characterized by lesions near mucosal membranes. The initial symptom of infection is a small red papule that ulcerates in a few weeks. The lesions are flat (no raised rim) and often oozing. Infections of the ear, nose and mouth area lead to degeneration of the cartilage and soft tissues resulting in disfigurement.

Transmission

Leishmaniasis is transmitted through the bites of infected female *Phlebotomine* sandflies. The epidemiology of leishmaniasis depends on the characteristics of the parasite species, the local ecological characteristics of the transmission sites, current and past exposure of the human population to the parasite and human behaviour. In South-East Asia, including India, *Visceral leishmaniasis* is the main form of the disease. Transmission generally occurs in rural areas below 600m above sea level with a heavy annual rainfall, a mean humidity above 70%, and a temperature range of 15-38°C, abundant vegetation, subsoil water and alluvial soil. The disease is most common in agricultural villages where houses are frequently constructed with mud walls and earthen floors, and cattle and other livestock live in close proximity to humans. In India including the state of Bihar only *Visceral leishmaniasis*, i.e. Kala-Azar is prevalent and there is only one anthroponotic reservoir, i.e. man for the disease transmission.

Ecology (Including Pathogenesis)

L. donovani spends the first portion of its life cycle living symbiotically in a sandfly and the second half of its life cycle living in the lymphatic system, vascular system, bone marrow, liver, and spleen of humans. The organism causes disease in humans by destroying host cells in the affected parts of the body causing abnormal enlargement of the target organs among other symptoms. Other symptoms of this disease can include a prolonged fever, a decreased appetite, weight loss, signs of anaemia, abdominal distension, and abnormal enlargement of the spleen and liver. Coughing, darkening of the skin, chronic diarrhoea, infection of the lymph nodes, and signs of chronic kidney disease may also by symptomatic of *Visceral leishmaniasis*.

Post-Kala-Azar Dermal Leishmaniasis (PKDL)

Post-Kala-Azar dermal leishmaniasis (PKDL) is a late complication of *Visceral leishmaniasis* (*VL*), which usually appears several months after treatment of a *VL* episode. PKDL is seen in areas where *L. donovani* is endemic i.e. in India. PKDL is characterized by a spectrum of skin lesions ranging from hypo-pigmented macules, papules to nodules or combinations over the trunk and face that can be easily confused with other skin conditions such as vitiligo or leprosy. PKDL accounts for about 5-10% of *Visceral leishmaniasis* in India. Both PKDL and *VL* are caused by *Leishmania amastogotes*, which are the commonest causative organism for Kala-Azar in India. PKDL is seen in about 10% of Kala-Azar patients in our country. It usually appears six months to one or more years after Kala-Azar has apparently been cured. But it can occur earlier. People with PKDL are considered to be a potential source of Kala-Azar infection. It is presumed that skin lesions of a late sequel of the visceral form called post-kala-azar-dermal leishmanisis (PKDL) act as reservoirs.

Intracellular Mechanism of Infection

The strategy of the pathogens like *Leishmania* to avoid destruction by the immune system and to thrive is just by 'hiding' itself inside a cell. This location enables it to avoid the action of the humoral immune response (because the pathogen is safely inside a cell and outside the open bloodstream), and furthermore it may prevent the immune system from destroying its host through non-danger surface signals which discourage apoptosis. The primary cell types *Leishmania* infiltrates the phagocytotic cells such as neutrophils and macrophages. Usually, a phagocytotic immune cell like a macrophage will ingest a pathogen within an enclosed endosome and then fill this endosome with enzymes which digest the pathogen.

However, in the case of *Leishmania*, these enzymes have no effect allowing the parasite to multiply rapidly. This uninhibited growth of parasites eventually overwhelms the host macrophage or other immune cell, causing it to die.

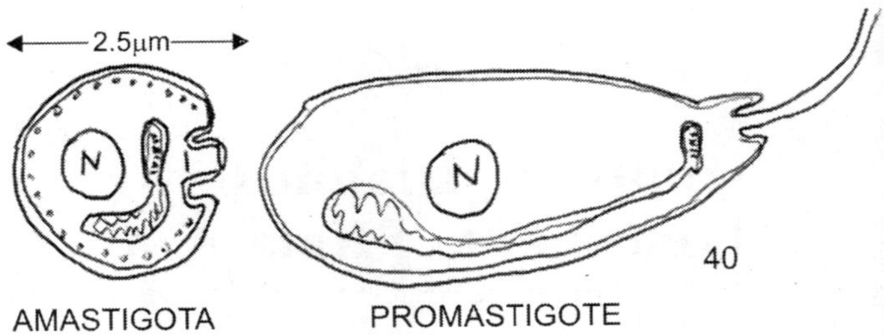

Fig. 9.

□

5

Symptoms, Diagnosis and Treatment of Kala-Azar

Kala-Azar is characterized by typical signs and symptoms which include:

- Recurrent fever intermittent or remittent with often double rise
- Loss of appetite, pallor and weight loss with progressive emaciation
- Weakness
- Splenomegaly-spleen enlarges rapidly causing massive enlargement usually soft and non-tender
- Liver enlargement not to the extent of spleen with soft and smooth surface along with sharp edge.

Lymphadenopathy – Not Very Common in India

- Skin – dry, thin and scaly and hair may be lost. Light-coloured persons show greyish discolouration on the skin of hands, feet, abdomen and face which gives the Indian name Kala-Azar meaning "Black fever".
- Anaemia develops rapidly. Anaemia with emaciation and gross splenomegaly produces a typical appearance of the patients.

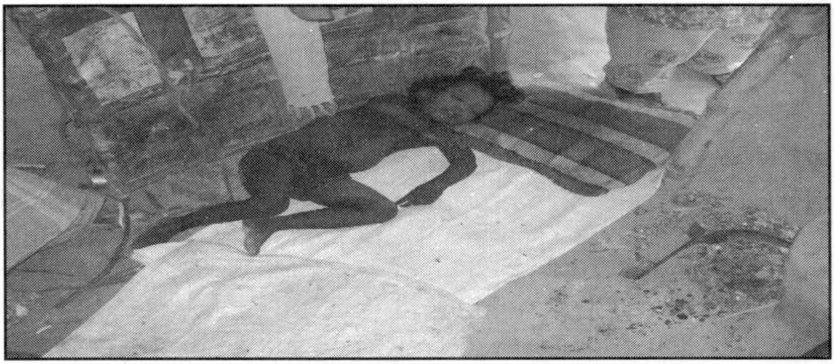

Fig. 10. Typical presentation of Kala-Azar.

The clinical and epidemiological findings in various forms of leishmaniasis are non-pathognomonic and these can mimic several other conditions. Hence, a laboratory diagnosis is required to confirm the clinical suspicion. The diagnostic tools used for each leishmanial syndrome, viz. *Visceral*, *Cutaneous*, and *Mucocutaneous* forms vary but the gold standard in each case remains to be the demonstration and isolation of the parasite from appropriate tissues.

Parasitological Diagnosis

The diagnosis of leishmaniasis is reliably made by the demonstration of the parasite in smears and by isolation either in culture or by animal inoculation of a biopsy sample or tissue aspirate from the spleen, or the bone marrow. The sensitivity is highest for splenic aspiration (as high as 98%) but so is the risk of complications such as haemorrhage. Occasionally, the amastigotes have also been demonstrated in liver biopsy (50-85% sensitive), lymph node aspirates and buffy coat smears particularly in HIV-Leishmania co-infection cases.

Serological Diagnosis

Conventional smear or culture techniques have low sensitivity particularly in detecting the occult and subclinical infections. These techniques are also cumbersome, time consuming and not suitable for field. The serological diagnosis is based on the presence of specific humoral response as in cases of *Visceral leishmaniasis* or cell-mediated immune response or *Cutaneous* and *Mucocutaneous leishmaniasis*. A wide range of serological methods varying in sensitivity and specificity are available for the diagnosis of *VL*. These serological methods can be grouped into non-specific and specific tests.

The non-specific tests had been in use in the past but are very rarely used these days. A positive test does not confirm the diagnosis of *Leishmaniasis*. Indirect hemagglutination (IHA), counter-current immune-electrophoresis (CCIEP), and Immuno-diffusion (ID) are examples of non-specific tests. These tests are cumbersome and have lower sensitivity and specificity and hence not commonly used. Some more commonly used ones are described below.

Leishmanin Skin Test (LST)

Delayed hypersensitivity is an important feature of cutaneous forms of human leishmaniasis and can be measured by the leishmanin test, also known as the Montenegro reaction. Leishmanin is a killed suspension of whole (0.5-1 × 10/ml) or disrupted (250 μg protein/ml) promastigotes in pyrogen-free phenol saline.

Leishmanin Skin Test is usually used as an indicator of the prevalence of *Cutaneous* and *Mucocutaneous leishmaniasis* in human and animal populations and successful cure of *Visceral leishmaniasis*. During active Kala-Azar disease, there will be no or negligible cell mediated immune response. However, the leishmanin antigen is not commercially available and no field study has been carried out in India.

Indirect Fluorescent Antibody Test (IFAT)

The Indirect Fluorescent Antibody Test is one of the

most sensitive available tests. The test is based on detecting antibodies which are demonstrated at the very early stages of infection and remain undetectable for six to nine months after cure. If the antibodies persist in low titres, it is good indication of a probable relapse. Titres above 1:20 are significant and above 1:128 are diagnostic. There is a possibility of a cross reaction with trypanosomal sera. However, this can be overcome by using leishmania amastigotes as an antigen instead of the promastigotes. Although this test is more sensitive (96%) and specific (98%) than soluble antigen ELISA, it is cumbersome and not suitable for field conditions.

Direct Agglutination Test

The Direct Agglutination Test (DAT) is a highly specific and sensitive test. It is inexpensive and simple to perform making it ideal for both field and laboratory use. The method uses whole stained promastigotes either as a suspension or in a freeze-dried form. The freeze-dried form is heat stable and facilitates the use of DAT in the field. However, the major disadvantage of DAT is the relatively long incubation time of 18 hrs and the need for serial dilutions of serum. Also, DAT has no prognostic value. The test may remain positive for several years after cure. Recently, Schoone et al. has developed a Fast Agglutination Screening Test (FAST) for the rapid detection (<three hours) of anti-leishmania antibodies in serum samples and on blood collected on filter paper.

The FAST utilises only one serum dilution leading to qualitative results. It offers the advantages of DAT based on the freeze-dried antigen, reproducibility, specificity and sensitivity of the antigen. Direct agglutination test has been evaluated for the diagnosis of *Cutaneous leishmaniasis* using L. major promastigotes and was shown to be highly specific and sensitive (90.5%).

Enzyme-Linked Immuno-Sorbent Assay

The Enzyme-Linked Immuno-Sorbent Assay (ELISA) is a valuable tool in the serodiagnosis of leishmaniasis. The test is useful for laboratory analysis as well as for field applications. However, the sensitivity and specificity of ELISA is greatly influenced by the antigen used. More recently, several recombinant antigens like rGBP from *L. donovani*, rORFF from *L. infantum*, rgp63, rK9, rK26 and rK39 from *L. chagasi* have been developed and tested. Of these, the rK39 antigen is found to be highly sensitive and predictive of onset of disease manifestation in *VL* patients.

In contrast, it does not show detectable antibodies in *Cutaneous* or *Mucocutaneous* leishmaniasis. The antibody titres to this antigen directly correlate with active disease and have potential in monitoring the chemotherapy and in predicting the clinical relapse. In addition rK39 ELISA has a high predictive value for detecting *VL* in immune-compromised persons, like those with AIDS. A kit (InBios®, USA) using this antigen and based on lateral flow is now commercially available in the form of antigen-impregnated nitrocellulose paper strips adapted for use under field conditions. The rK39 strip test has been found highly sensitive and a reliable indicator of Kala-Azar in India.

Immunoblotting

Most of the work concerning the use of immunoblotting in the diagnosis of leishmaniasis has been done on *VL*. In cutaneous leishmaniasis, anti-leishmania antibodies though detectable are present in low titres. Hence, immunoblotting is not widely adopted for diagnosing *CL*. The biggest advantage of immunoblotting, as a general rule, is that various antigens expressed and antibodies recognised during the course of infection can be documented. It also has an added advantage of permanent documentation.

However, the technique is not user-friendly and is limited only to research laboratories. Though a few reports are published, no satisfactory antigen detection system is currently available. Recently, a latex agglutination test (KATEX) for the detection of leishmanial antigens in the urine of patients with *VL* has been developed. The results obtained with KATEX using samples collected from patients of different foci of *VL* indicate that the test works well regardless of the geographical origin of samples. The test had 100% specificity and sensitivity between 68-100%. Whether the test has applications for the detection of asymptomatic cases of *VL* and monitoring therapy is yet to be confirmed. There are no antigen detection systems currently available for *CL* and *MCL*.

Molecular Methods

Microscopy and culture have the limitations of low sensitivity and are time consuming. The immunological methods fail to distinguish between past and present infections and are not very reliable in immune-compromised patients. While the molecular approach is capable of detecting nucleic acids unique to the parasite, it would address these limitations. A variety of nucleic acid detection methods targeting both DNA and RNA have been developed. Amongst these the PCR has proved to be a highly sensitive and specific technique. The PCR assay can detect parasite DNA or RNA a few weeks ahead of appearance of any clinical signs or symptoms. Different DNA sequences in the genome of leishmania like ITS region, gp63 locus, telomeric sequences, sequence targets in rRNA genes such as 18s rRNA and SSU-rRNA and both conserved and variable regions in kinetoplast DNA (kDNA) minicircles are being used by various workers.

Summary of Diagnostic Methods in Indian Context

Demonstration of parasites is the most reliable and

conventional method for diagnosing *VL*. The parasite is commonly found in the splenic or bone marrow aspirate and in the buffy coat of peripheral blood (in HIV co-infection). The sensitivity of splenic aspirate smear is more than 95% and is regarded as the gold standard for the diagnosis of Kala-Azar. Splenic aspiration carries the risk of severe haemorrhage. The sensitivity of bone marrow smear (the other diagnostic option) is only about 60-85% and the procedure is quite painful. Although several Serodiagnostic tests have been developed, e.g. ELISA and IFAT, yet none is in practice because of drawbacks like high cost, need for electricity, complicated technical procedures and unsatisfactory specificity and sensitivity. Direct agglutination test is a cheap, sensitive and specific test and is popular in Africa, but it is associated with drawbacks like batch-to-batch variation, instability of the antigen, need for incubation and a cumbersome procedure, and thus is not popular in India. In Bihar, rk39 is the only current method of diagnosing Kala-Azar.

Treatment: The treatment guidelines in India are represented as below:

Table 1: Treatment Guidelines for Kala-Azar in India

Drug	**Remarks**	**Dosages**
Injection SSG	1st line drug treatment	20 mg. per kg. body weight daily for 20 days. Maximum 8.5 ml per day
Injection Amphotericin-B	2nd line drug treatment	1 mg. per kg. body weight alternate days (15 injections)
Capsule Miltefosine	2nd line drug treatment	50 mg. below 12 years; 100 mg. above 12 years; 2.5 mg. 1 kg body weight (56 tablets) for 28 days (adult dose)

The treatment options for *Visceral leishmaniasis* are limited and far from satisfactory. Pentavalent antimonials (sodium stibogluconate; SbV) and Amphotericin B (Amp B) have been the two drugs with proven efficacy for treatment of *VL*. Both the drugs are given parenterally and are potentially toxic. Paromomycin, an aminoglycoside antibiotic, is currently undergoing Phase-III clinical trial. Recently, for the first time anoral antileishmanial drug "Miltefosine" has proved effective in treating Indian *VL* and has been registered for treatment of *VL*. Miltefosine has been rolled out in 16 highly endemic districts of Bihar.

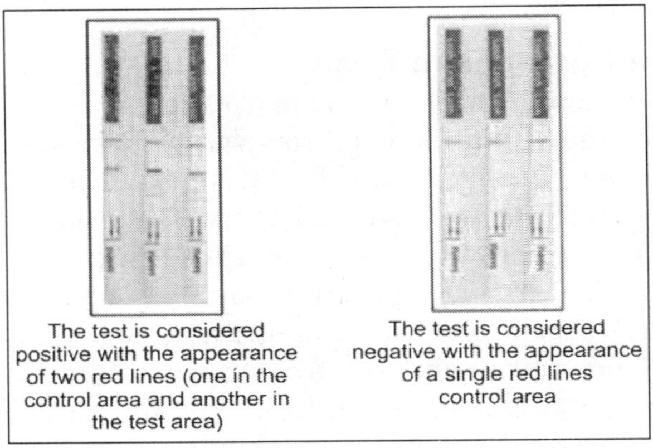

Fig. 11. rk 39 diagnostic kit for kala-azar

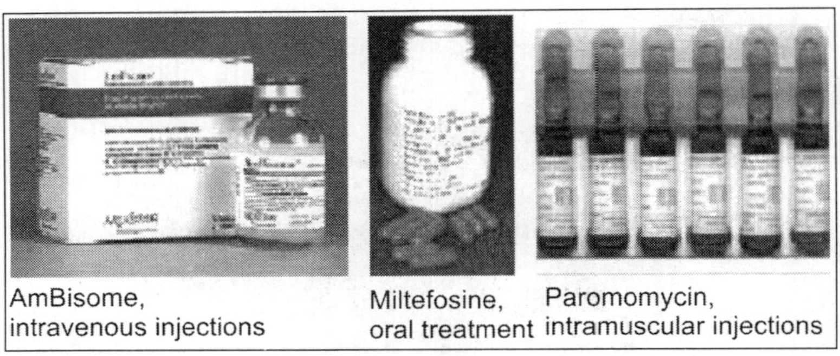

Fig. 12. Drugs for Kala-Azar treatment

□

6

Epidemiology of Kala-Azar

Disease Patterns in Bihar

Kala-Azar Control Programme is nationally sponsored under National Vector-Borne Disease Control Programme (NVBDCP), by the Ministry of Health and Family Welfare, Govt. of India. However, the surveillance of Kala-Azar is under the Integrated Disease Surveillance programme (IDSP), which is one of its flagship programmes. The surveillance programme focuses on control and management of communicable diseases including Kala-Azar through three types of surveillance, viz. Presumptive, Laboratory and Syndromic surveillance.

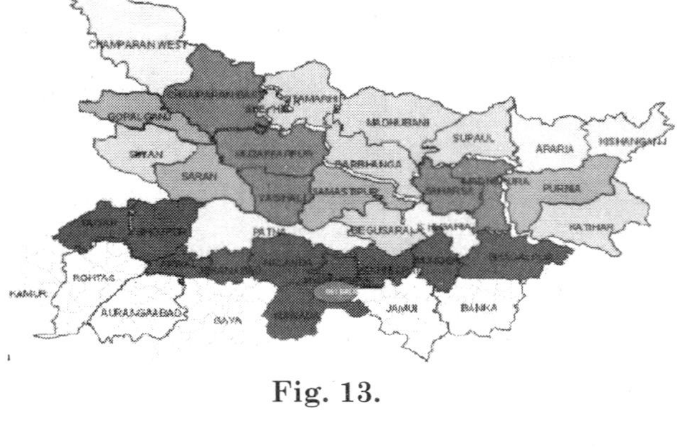

Fig. 13.

Endemicity of Kala-Azar in Bihar

The map shows different colours as per incidence of the disease. Red-coloured areas are districts with highest incidence followed by green, orange and yellow. Blue-coloured areas are places with lower incidence but are relatively new for the disease spreads. Outbreaks have been reported in these new areas which is a matter of grave concern.

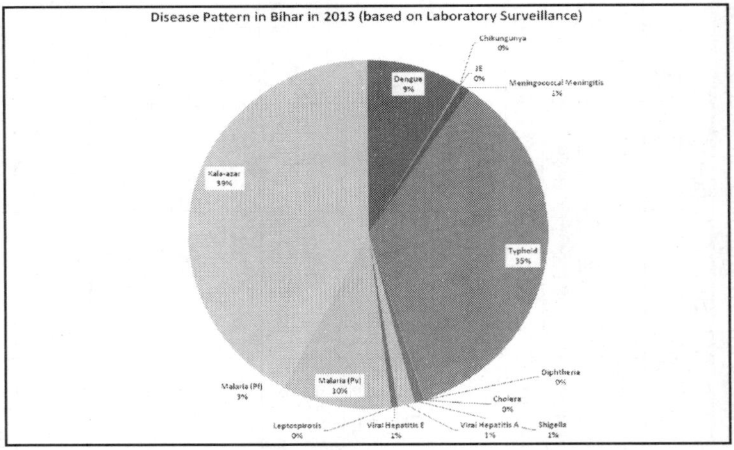

Fig. 14. Disease Pattern in Bihar in 2013.

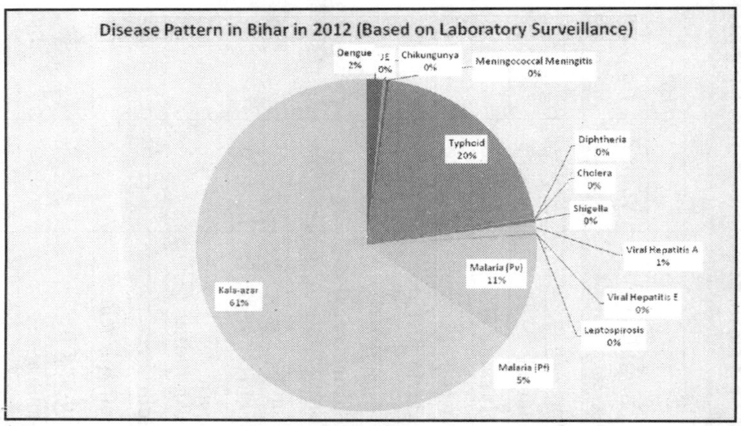

Fig. 15. Disease Pattern in Bihar in 2012.

Table 2: Number and Proportion of Cases for all Reportable Diseases in Bihar by Ranking (Based on Lab Surveillance)

Reportable Diseases	*2010*		*2011*		*2012*		*2013*	
	Number of Cases	*Proportion of Cases(%)*	*Number of Cases*	*Proportion of Cases(%)*	*Number of Cases*	*Proportion of Cases(%)*	*Number of Cases*	*Proportion of Cases(%)*
Kala-Azar	23084	87	25009	81	13797	61	9929	39
Typhoid	875	3.3	2390	8	4571	20	9088	35.4
Malaria (Pv)	560	2.1	1549	5	2373	10	2505	10
Dengue	1125	4.2	46	0.14	350	2	2206	9
Malaria (Pf)	528	2	1075	4	1029	5	888	3.4
Viral Hepatitis A	91	0.34	142	0.46	239	1	389	2
Meningococcal Meningitis	59	0.22	118	0.38	63	0.27	219	0.85
Shigella	59	0.22	118	0.38	89	0.4	220	0.85
Viral Hepatitis E	0	0	5	0.01	22	0.09	152	0.59
Japanese Encephalitis (JE)	0	0	159	0.5	63	0.27	37	0.14
Diphtheria	0	0	2	0.006	23	0.01	17	0.06
Leptospirosis	0	0	2	0.006	6	0.02	7	0.02
Chikungunya	0	0	80	0.26	10	0.04	4	0.01
Cholera	20	0.07	0	0	0	0	0	0
Total	**26401**	**100**	**30695**	**100**	**22635**	**100**	**25661**	**100**

The disease proportion has been calculated on the basis of laboratory surveillance. 14 reportable diseases are included under laboratory surveillance under the Integrated Disease Surveillance Programme in the State.

Spread of Kala-Azar at a Glance

In Bihar, 33 districts out of 38 are endemic for Kala-Azar. Out of these, 11 most affected districts are Vaishali, Saran, Muzaffarpur, Darbhangha, W. Champaran, Sitamarhi, Araria, Purnea, Sahharsa, Madhepura and Samastipur, which involve 80% of the overall reported Kala-Azar cases in Bihar. Sheikhpura district was affected with the disease when 58 cases were reported in 2011. The number of cases of Kala-Azar has shown decline in 2013. The proportion of Kala-Azar cases out of total reported cases has reduced from 61% in 2012 to 39% in 2013. This is a good news and may partly be due to the camp-based search of new cases and proper case management. In 2013, Kala-Azar cases were reported from only 28 districts out of 33 endemic districts. There is provisioning of diagnosis and treatment of Kala-Azar patients in all sadar hospitals, sub-divisional hospitals, referral hospitals and PHCs of the affected districts.

The treatment is done with three types of drugs, viz. SAG, Miltefosine and Amphotericin B. In Vaishali district, NGOs are providing treatment with Ambisome in five most affected PHCs viz. Raghopur, Vaishali, Mahua, Bidupur and Garaul. The Health Department of the State provides ₹ 50/- a day to Kala-Azar patients (upto maximum of 30 days) to compensate the loss of wages. In all Govt. Hospitals, free food is provided to Kala-Azar patient and his one attendant during the treatment process. In rural areas, ASHA workers are provided incentive of ₹ 200 for each Kala-Azar case searched, identified and treated patients. To aware the community regarding Kala-Azar and its control, IEC and

IPC activities are being undertaken that involves printing of posters and handbills regarding involvement of community in DDT spray. The display of hoardings related to Kala-Azar at public places is also being undertaken. Epidemiological analysis of the data reveals that the male population (60.25%) is more affected with the disease than females (39.75%).

The age group most affected includes: 11-20>0-10>21-30>31-40>51-60>61+. This interpretation should be kept in mind while adopting and applying treatment regimens as the recent analysis shows that incidence of Kala-Azar is rising in children, particularly of the age group 0-10 years and youngsters of the age group 11-20.

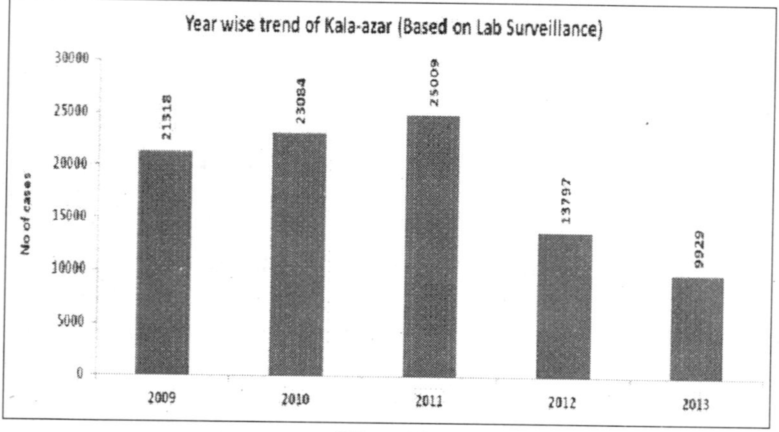

Fig. 16.

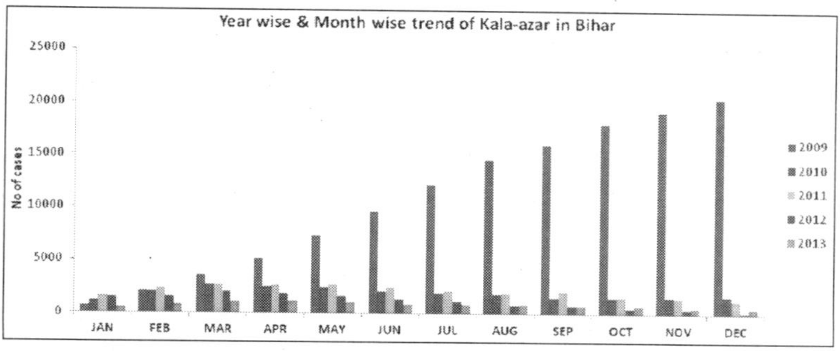

Fig. 17.

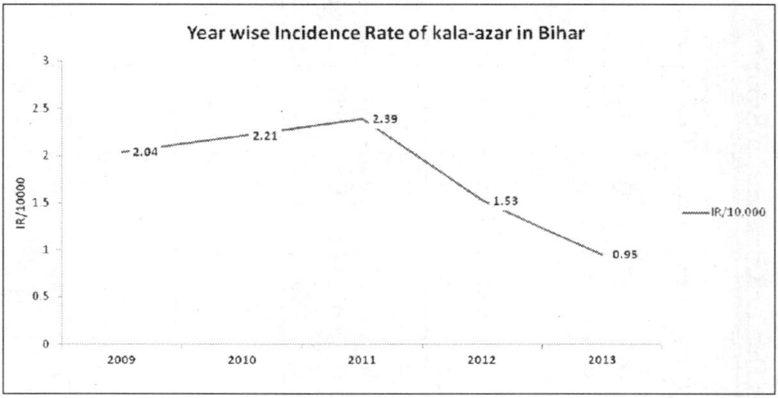
Year wise Incidence Rate of kala-azar in Bihar
IR/10000
2.04
2.21
2.39
1.53
0.95
IR/10,000
2009
2010
2011
2012
2013

Fig. 18.

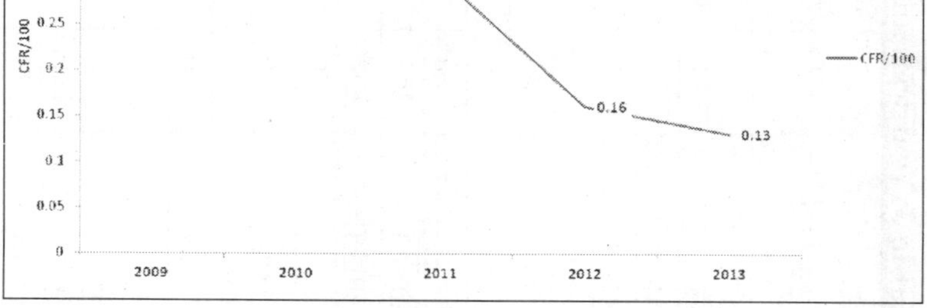
Year wise Case Fatality Rate due to Kala-azar in Bihar
CFR/100
0.37
0.41
0.3
0.16
0.13
CFR/100
2009
2010
2011
2012
2013

Fig. 19.

Table 3: Year-wise and District-wise Cases and Deaths Due to Kala-Azar in Bihar

		2013		*2012*		*2011*		*2010*		*2009*	
S. No.	*District*	*Cases*	*Deaths*	*Cases*	*Deaths*	*Cases*	*Deaths*	*Cases*	*Deaths*	*Cases*	*Deaths*
1.	Araria	746	0	907	0	1716	0	2037	0	1575	3
2.	Arwal	2	0	3	0	1	0	2	0	2	0
3.	Aurangabad	0	0	0	0	0	0	0	0	0	0
4.	Banka	2	0	7	0	1	0	0	0	2	0
5.	Begusarai	246	0	310	0	328	2	293	5	272	4
6.	Bhagalpur	66	0	128	1	170	4	105	4	47	2
7.	Bhojpur	0	0	7	0	21	0	15	0	7	0
8.	Buxar	5	0	14	0	14	0	10	0	50	2
9.	Darbhanga	451	0	696	0	1121	0	1019	0	947	1
10.	E. Champaran	702	4	1021	2	1399	6	1280	14	1365	5
11.	Gaya	0	0	0	0	0	0	0	0	0	0
12.	Gopalganj	486	0	512	0	930	0	877	0	767	0
13.	Jamui	0	0	0	0	0	0	0	0	0	0
14.	Jehanabad	0	0	20	0	20	0	14	0	19	0
15.	Kaimur	0	0	0	2	0	0	0	0	0	0
16.	Katihar	454	1	615	0	927	8	708	8	532	5
17.	Khagaria	199	0	275	0	324	0	329	0	309	0
18.	Kishanganj	174	0	144	0	222	0	167	0	128	1

19. Lakhisarai	17	0	21	0	62	0	15	0	5	0
20. Madhepura	481	0	651	3	1520	4	1721	3	1591	3
21. Madhubani	321	2	422	0	543	2	630	2	732	2
22. Munger	91	0	54	0	104	2	60	1	40	1
23. Muzaffarpur	1061	4	1618	6	2782	18	2573	22	2329	11
24. Nalanda	15	0	24	1	18	0	11	0	13	2
25. Nawada	0	0	7	0	32	0	17	0	61	4
26. Patna	140	0	122	2	170	3	141	4	133	2
27. Purnea	764	1	1387	0	2232	1	2238	8	2138	1
28. Rohtas	0	0	0	0	0	0	0	0	0	0
29. Saharsa	837	0	1146	1	2191	4	2230	5	2150	5
30. Samastipur	484	0	838	0	1233	2	1261	1	1158	3
31. Saran	646	0	1069	1	1733	4	1103	1	1055	2
32. Sheikhpura	0	0	20	1	58	1	0	0	0	0
33. Sheohar	0	0	180	0	213	0	95	0	110	0
34. Sitamarhi	0	0	826	4	1294	12	934	8	726	15
35. Siwan	454	0	628	1	786	0	715	1	660	0
36. Supaul	154	1	236	0	320	0	396	0	386	1
37. Vaishali	862	0	2076	2	2421	3	1989	7	1883	4
38. W. Champaran	69	0	72	0	103	0	99	1	126	1
TOTAL	**9929**	**13**	**16056**	**27**	**25009**	**76**	**23084**	**95**	**21318**	**80**

Table 4: No. of Kala-Azar Affected PHCs in Bihar in 2013

Sl. No.	*District Affected*	*No. of PHCs*
1.	Araria	9
2.	Aurangabad	0
3.	Arwal	2
4.	Banka	2
5.	Begusarai	17
6.	Bhagalpur	11
7.	Bhojpur	4
8.	Buxar	3
9.	Darbhangha	15
10.	E. Champaran	20
11.	Gaya	0
12.	Gopalganj	13
13.	Jamui	0
14.	Jahanabad	2
15.	Kaimur	0
16.	Katihar	17
17.	Khagaria	7
18.	Kishanganj	7
19.	Lakhisarai	5
20.	Madhepura	13
21.	Madhubani	19
22.	Munger	3
23.	Muzaffarpur	16
24.	Nawada	0
25.	Nalanda	5
26.	Patna	24
27.	Purnia	14
28.	Rohtas	0
29.	Saharsa	10
30.	Samastipur	19
31.	Saran	15
32.	Sheikhpura	1
33.	Sheohar	5
34.	Sitamarhi	16
35.	Siwan	19
36.	Supaul	9
37.	Vaishali	16
38.	W. Champaran	10
	Total	**348**

Table 5: Comparative Analysis of Incidence Rate (IR) of Kala-Azar/10,000 Population in Bihar (on the Basis of Increasing Incidence rate in Respective Years)

	2013		*2012*		*2011*		*2010*		*2009*	
Sl. No.	*District*	*IR/ 10,000*	*District*	*IR/ 10,000*	*District*	*IR/ 10,000*	*District*	*IR/ 10,000*	*District*	*IR/ 10,000*
1.	Saharsa	4.19	Vaishali	6.24	Saharsa	10.98	Saharsa	11.2	Saharsa	10.8
2.	Araria	2.65	Saharsa	5.74	Madhepura	7.75	Madhepura	8.77	Madhepura	8.11
3.	Vaishali	2.59	Purnea	4.04	Vaishali	7.28	Araria	7.24	Purnea	6.23
4.	Madhepura	2.45	Madhepura	3.32	Purnea	6.51	Purnea	6.52	Vaishali	5.7
5.	Muzaffarpur	2.3	Araria	3.22	Araria	6.1	Vaishali	5.98	Araria	5.6
6.	Purnea	2.2	Saran	2.72	Saran	4.42	Muzaffarpur	5.59	Gopalganj	3

Comparative Analysis of Case Fatality Rate (CFR) of Kala-Azar/100 in Bihar (on the Basis of Increasing CFR in Respective Years)

	2013		*2012*		*2011*		*2010*		*2009*	
Sl. No.	*District*	*CFR/ 100*	*District*	*CFR/ 100*	*District*	*CFR/ 100*	*District*	*CFR/ 100*	*District*	*CFR/ 100*
1.	Supaul	0.64	Sheikhpura	5	Bhagalpur	2.35	Bhagalpur	3.8	Nalanda	15.38
2.	Madhubani	0.62	Nalanda	4.16	Munger	1.92	Patna	2.83	Nawada	6.55
3.	E. Champaran	0.56	Patna	1.63	Patna	1.76	Begusarai	1.7	Bhagalpur	4.25
4.	Muzaffarpur	0.37	Bhagalpur	0.78	Sheikhpura	1.72	Munger	1.66	Munger	2.5
5.	Katihar	0.22	Sitamarhi	0.48	Sitamarhi	0.92	Katihar	1.12	Sitamarhi	2.06
6.	Purnea	0.13	Madhepura	0.46	Begusarai	0.6	W Champaran	1.01	Patna	1.5

Table 6: List of PHCs Showing Highest Incidence Rate (IR)/10,000 for Kala-Azar in Endemic Districts of Bihar in 2013

Sl. No.	*District*	*PHC*	*IR/10,000*
1.	Araria	Raniganj	7.2
		Araria	4.7
		Kurshakanta	4.42
2.	Arwal	Kurtha	0.07
		Arwal	0.06
3.	Banka	Fulidumar	0.07
		Chanan	0.05
4.	Begusarai	Dandari	4.09
		Bachwara	1.86
		Kodabandpur	1.42
5.	Bhagalpur	Pir-Paiti	0.75
		Kahalgaon	0.52
		Rangra	0.3
6.	Bhojpur	Barhara	0.15
		Udvant Nagar	0.14
		Koilwar	0.09
7.	Buxar	Buxar	0.1
		Nawanagar	0.048
		Brahmpur	0.041
8.	Darbhangha	K Asthan	3.51
		Jally	1.94
		Hayaghat	1.77
9.	E. Champaran	Chakiya	3.59
		Kasariya	3.52
		Turkauliya	3.14
10.	Gopalganj	Barauli	4.19
		Manjha	3.11
		Baikunthpur	2.99
11.	Jehanabad	Kako	0.11
		Jahanabad	0.07

12.	Katihar	Hasanganj	8.39
		Pranpur	4.88
		Sameli	4.4
13.	Khagaria	Beldaur	2.87
		Alauli	2.5
		Gogri	1.23
14.	Kishanganj	Dighalbank	2.2
		Bahadurganj	1.89
		Thakurganj	1.4
15.	Lakhisarai	Pipariya	0.77
		Surajgarha	0.32
		Ramgarh	0.11
16.	Madhepura	Ghamharia	5.02
		Ghailar	3.79
		UDA Kishanganj	3.58
17.	Madhubani	Bisfi	1.58
		Jaynagar	1.26
		Jhanjharpur	1.07
18.	Munger	Bariyarpur	6.96
		Jamalpur	0.25
		Haveli Kharagpur	0.11
19.	Muzaffarpur	Sahabganj	4.99
		Bandra	4.37
		Paroo	3.87
20.	Nawada	NIL cases	NIL cases
21.	Nalanda	Parwarpur	0.41
		Nagaunaussa	0.33
		Silaw	0.13
22.	Patna	Athmalgola	1.68
		Dhanarua	1.3
		Vikram	0.52
23.	Purnea	Shri Nagar	4.66
		K. Nagar	4.3

		B. Koti	3.98
24.	Saharsa	Sour Bazar	9.82
		Simri Bakhtiarpur	5.85
		Salkhua	5.47
25.	Samastipur	Warisnagar	2.45
		Sarai Ranjan	2.23
		Bithan	1.98
26.	Saran	Baniyapur	2.58
		Amnaur	2.35
		Mashrakh	2.28
27.	Shekhpura	Sheikpura	0.41
28.	Sheohar	Dumri Katsari	2.85
		Piprahi	2.56
		Sheohar	2.04
29.	Sitamarhi	Parsauni	6.69
		Bathanaha	3.15
		Bejapatti	2.8
30.	Siwan	Basantpur	6.68
		Nautan	4.52
		Goria Kothi	3.95
31.	Supaul	Raghopur	2.05
		Supaul	1.32
		Pipra	0.93
32.	Vaishali	Raghopur	6.98
		Mahua	3.84
		Mahnar	2.71
33.	W. Champaran	Thakraha	1.53
		Majhaulia	0.67
		Nautan	0.44

□

7

Kala-Azar Control Strategy

Kala-Azar has been endemic in India since long. Earlier outbreaks occurred in the early nineteenth century, which used to occur in cyclical epidemics at the intervals of 10-15 years. However, the disease declined to negligible proportions during 1953 and 1958.

Kala-Azar Elimination by 2015

Insecticide Residual Spray (IRS) with DDT in between 1953 and 1958 under National Malaria Eradication Programme resulted in marked decline in the disease incidence. Resurgence of Kala-Azar was noted in 1970s subsequent to withdrawal of IRS. In Bihar, Kala-Azar cases were reported from four districts and then from other parts as well. However, after reporting of 77102 cases and 1049 deaths in 1992, which were quite high, Government of India launched centrally-sponsored Kala-Azar Control Programme based on the recommendation of an expert committee to eliminate Kala-Azar by the year, 2000. Thereafter, National Health Policy set the goal for Kala-Azar elimination by 2010. Furthermore; a tripartite Memorandum of Understanding was signed between India, Bangladesh and Nepal for elimination of Kala-Azar by 2015. In Bihar, presently 33 districts are endemic for kala-azar.

Kala-Azar Control Programme is nationally sponsored under National Vector-Borne Disease Control Programme (NVBDCP), Ministry of Health and Family Welfare, Govt. of India. It is provided fund by Government of India. The surveillance of Kala-Azar is also focused under the Integrated Disease Surveillance Programme (IDSP) which is also a flagship programme of Ministry of Health and Family Welfare, Government of India. The surveillance Programme focuses on control and management of communicable diseases including Kala-Azar through three types of surveillance, viz. Presumptive, Laboratory and Syndromic surveillance.

Control of Kala-Azar is based on three-pronged strategy which includes:

1. Vector Control and Management
2. Parasite Elimination
3. Supporting Interventions

Vector Control and Management

It is an essential component as no vaccine or drug is available for the prevention and cure of Kala-Azar. It can be a combination of measures designed to prevent breeding of sandfly densities and measures to reduce the populations of the vector species. Vector management may be under taken in two ways:

One involving control measures during Kala-Azar outbreaks and the other involving control measures during inter-epidemic period.

During an outbreak, the control measures are targeted to reduce the load of infective vector species while during inter-epidemic periods, vector-control measures are mostly preventive designed to prevent the build-up of vector population beyond critical levels.

Components of Vector Management

Vector management is an important intervention for

control of kala-azar. Various components of vector management are briefed below:

(i) *Personal Protection:* This includes using protective clothing, mats, coils and aerosols and repellents.

(ii) *Habitat Management:* This includes the periodical cleaning and plastering of cracks in walls, floors, construction of *pucca* houses and removal of garbage, vegetation and collection of dung heaps, etc.

(iii) *Biological Control:* This includes use of predators or bio-larvicides – Bacillus formulation (B.t.i. or B.s.) in their natural breeding or resting places or fungi.

(iv) *Chemical Control:* This includes selective IRS in human dwelling and cattle sheds only when the vector population builds up above threshold level. Other methods include space spraying that involves the application of small droplets of insecticides into air in an attempt to kill vector, thermal or cold fogging which is resorted for vector control in emergency situations. It has limited effectiveness and should be restricted in routine use.

(v) *Environmental Management:* This involves any change that prevents or minimizes vector breeding and hence reduces human vector contact. Important component includes environmental modifications like use of long-lasting physical transformation of vector habitats, improved housing structure, proofing of human dwelling and sleeping on cots. Other component includes changes to human habitat or behaviour that includes efforts to reduce man-vector-parasite contact, use of impregnated bed nets, sleeping on cots or above the ground surface, staying away from cattle sheds, proper sanitation, and removal of any garbage near the house.

(vi) *Inter-sectoral coordination:* Inter-sectoral coordination is the key to control of kala-azar. Active community participation for vector control, spray activities, referral of patients with symptoms of Kala-Azar is required for successful control of Kala-Azar. Involvement of various sectors such as Panchayat, Irrigation, floods, agriculture, education, sanitation, forest, non-governmental agencies (NGOs), and private practitioners, etc. is necessary for management and control of the disease.

(vii) *Information, Education and Communication (IEC):* IEC is an important intervention for management and control of vector as well as for elimination of Kala-Azar. Major components include inter-personal communication through primary health-care infrastructure, printed publicity like pamphlets, advertisements, folders and booklets, etc., audio-visual communication channels including nukkad-nataks and orientation of opinion leaders, etc. Besides, observing a 'Kala-Azar-Fortnight' with effective IEC inputs and simultaneous detection and treatment campaign is expected to provide an impetus for the control of the disease.

(viii) Legislation: It is also an important component for Kala-Azar control. It includes detection facilities at sub-centre level, notification of all Kala-Azar cases at all levels including private clinics, same treatment schedule for all and follow-ups of the all patients for proper treatment with proper screening.

Options for Vector Control

(i) *Indoor Residual Spray (IRS):* Control of the vector

sandflies through IRS is highly amenable due to vector behaviour. There is a record that in India, DDT spray led to disappearance of Kala-Azar in sixties era in Tamil Nadu. In nineties, incidence was brought down by >70% (Bihar) within three years after spray activities. Entomological monitoring evidence has shown the effect of DDT on adult prevalence. IRS remains the most effective vector control option. Studies on vector density carried out by State Surveillance Unit, Bihar also confirmed that vector density was less in sprayed areas when compared to the non-sprayed areas.

(ii) *Insecticide Treated Nets (ITN):* These are generally recommended where IRS cannot be done. Available literature indicates effectiveness in some situation but also doubts on effectiveness in other situations. Review commission of WHO (Alexander and Maroli, 2003) on impact of ITNs indicates two African studies (thermophilic species) showing good effect and other two as not effective. Adequate information on ITN effect against *P. argentipes* (Hygrophilic species) in Asia is not available.

(iii) *Insecticidal Residual Spray for Kala-Azar Control:* Indoor residual spraying is most important intervention in achieving the interruption of transmission of diseases transmitted by Phlebotomine sandflies. In the 1950s, anti-malaria spraying under the National Malaria Control Programme (NMCP) and National Malaria Eradication Programme (1958) brought about a virtual cessation of Kala-Azar transmission in India. Indoor residual spraying has virtually eliminated Kala-Azar from north-eastern states of Assam, Meghalaya and Tripura, and smaller foci in Orissa and Tamil Nadu.

The target of Kala-Azar elimination programme is aimed at stopping of Kala-Azar transmission by the year 2015. Thus, it is imperative that all Kala-Azar villages, whether affected in past or at present, are treated with insecticidal sprays.

Important components for selecting targets for spray activities include:

(i) All villages within a PHC which reported Kala-Azar cases in the past five years.
(ii) All villages which reported cases during the year of spraying.
(iii) Villages which are free of kala-azar, but on search are found to contain cases conforming to the Kala-Azar case definition.

The dosage of DDT application is the same as that for anti-malarial spraying, i.e. 1 g/m^2 on the wall surface. The inside walls of huts and cattle shed are to be treated with the insecticide. Spraying is to be restricted to the six feet of the wall surface. Cattle sheds, and Kala-Azar positive and suspected houses are to be treated on priority. Spraying is usually started to coincide with the build-up of vector populations and before onset of Kala-Azar transmission.

The transmission season of Kala-Azar in India is from June to October. The build-up in the population of the vector *P. argentipes* starts in March. The effectiveness of DDT deposits lasts for about 10 weeks. Two rounds of spraying to control *P. argentipes* population are undertaken in Bihar, first in February/March and second in May/June. Two rounds of sprays are given for DDT to provide protection during the entire transmission season. Focal spray includes spray in 50 houses in an area from where one Kala-Azar case has been reported. DDT 50% still remains the insecticide of choice as vectors are still susceptible to DDT 50%. It is estimated that for single and two round of spray 37.5 and 75 MT of DDT per million population of DDT is required respectively. Thus, an average requirement of DDT per 5000 population (which is sub-centre population) for single and double round of DDT spray is 187.5 and 375 kg. respectively.

Limited literature is available on resistance of sandflies to DDT, although in some pockets resistance/tolerance has been reported. Malathion 5% wp is the next choice for IRS. In Nepal and Bangladesh, synthetic pyrethroids are being used.

Components of IRS: Some of the important components of IRS include:

Spray Operations

This involves calculation of requirements of insecticides, preparation of suspensions, and spray technique. Various pre- and post-spray activities are planned for successful control of the vector. Pre-spray activities include selection of the areas to be sprayed, getting the required quantities of insecticides and equipment, hiring and training of spray squads and informing the community. Post-spray activities includes routine maintenance of equipment and minor repairs, reports and records, transportation, safe handling and storage of insecticides and supervision of process and performance indicators.

Concurrent Supervision

Good and concurrent supervision is key for successful control of kala-azar. Various activities requiring concurrent supervision includes date of advance notification and maintenance of time table for spray operation, turn out of spray crew, nozzle tip discharge rate, conditions of spray pumps, preparation of insecticidal suspension, actual spray operation including the technique, speed and coverage, etc., extent of refusal to accept spray and the numbers and percentage of locked houses, maintenance of spray records, consumption of insecticide as determined by the quantity issued and stock in hand, date and time of checking of the squad by inspectors/supervisors and other supervisory personnel and their remarks, if any, arrangement for mopping up, future programme and time schedule, evidence of insecticidal deposit on sprayable surfaces particularly corners, walls up to six feet windows, etc., dispersal of the insecticide deposits on walls to verify uniformity of deposits, number of rooms in each house sprayed satisfactorily, partially and not at all, percentage of refusal and locked houses, factors responsible for not spraying any area as elicited through enquiries from the residents, factor responsible for high refusal rates, if any and action taken, attempts made for mopping up operation in the event of high refusal, extent of mud plastering on the walls, if any and other relevant matters. This activity if properly supervised is expected to provide an impetus for successful spray activities.

(2) *Parasite Elimination:* This is the second pronged strategy for Kala-Azar control. Parasite elimination is aided by proper diagnosis and case management. Under this, Kala-Azar rapid test-rk39 has been introduced for use at the peripheral level. With the reporting of side effects of SAG and Amp B, oral drug Miltefosin has been introduced as first line treatment drug. Besides these strengthening of referral services by involvement of ASHAs has also been introduced.

(3) *Supporting Interventions:* This is third pronged strategy for Kala-Azar control. It involves various aspects like communication for behaviour impact, inter-sectoral collaboration, capacity building, operational research and close monitoring and supervision with periodic reviews/ evaluations.

Herbal Control: Future in Kala-Azar Control???

Vector control is the best method for control of the disease *Visceral leishmaniasis*. Synthetic chemical insecticides such as DDT, Malathion, Parathion, etc. have been used by the government bodies under the spay programme. Sandfly control programme in most *Visceral leishmaniasis* (*VL*)/Kalal-azar foci have advanced slowly when compared to other haematophagous insects like mosquitoes, ticks and black flies (Mutinga, 1992). This may be attributed due to the presence of sandflies in the areas where the mosquitoes also thrive. Thus, although *VL* is a serious disease, the main focus has been on the control of mosquito-borne diseases.

During 1950s and 1960s, anti-malaria control campaign utilizing residual DDT spray led to transient disappearance of sandflies and Kala-Azar in India, Pakistan and Bangladesh. This success was believed to be due to susceptibility of sandflies to DDT. Similar success was also seen in Italy, Greece, Russia and Israel where control of other forms of leishmaniasis were also achieved. In the Indian subcontinent because of the environmental and bio-accumulative effects of DDT, cessation of its use led to progressive resurgence of Kala-Azar including cases of post Kala-Azar dermal leishmaniasis (PKDL). Resistance in sandflies against the synthetic insecticides like DDT was also reported by (Pillai, 1996).

Present Status of Kala-Azar and Chemical Control in India

Visceral leishmaniasis has been a serious public health problem in the country since 1970s, in the State of Bihar that later spread to West Bengal and eastern Uttar Pradesh. In 1977, according to a sample survey estimate, about one lakh cases and 4500 deaths were reported in Bihar. The disease was initially prevalent in 31 districts in the State of Bihar (old Bihar). However, the Kala-Azar foci spread to two more districts, viz. Nawada and Sheikhpura leading to total of 33 affected districts in Bihar at present.

National Malaria Control Programme was launched in 1953, the same was later named as National Malaria Eradication Programme (NMEP) and at present it has been incorporated and merged under the National Vector- Borne Disease Control Programmes. Under this programme, DDT has been extensively used for control of vector sandflies as well as mosquitoes. The DDT spray operation reduced the sandfly population to the very low levels resulting in interruption of Kala-Azar transmission and virtual elimination of the disease. Spraying of residual insecticide was withdrawn under NMEP in a phased manner from different areas from 1962 onwards. In 1970s, Kala-Azar cases were again reported from Muzaffarpur, Sitamahari and Samastipur in Bihar. Kala-Azar incidence started showing increasing trend after resurgence till 1992. However, in last two years, viz. 2012 and 2013, Kala-Azar cases have showed drassic and abrupt decline by half.

Until 1989-490, Kala-Azar control activities were undertaken by the states on focal basis diverting NMEP resources. However, during 1990-91 Planning Commission approved a centrally-sponsored Kala-Azar Control Scheme in both the endemic states, namely Bihar and West Bengal. After the implementation of this scheme, Kala-Azar cases showed a sharp decline from 1993 and continued till 1999. However, in 2000 number of cases again increased significantly to 12964 with 202 deaths (data obtained from Bihar Directorate of Health Services).

In 2000, a multi-centric study was initiated by the Indian Council of Medical Research (ICMR) and Rajendra Memorial Research Institute of Medical Sciences (RMRIMS), Patna which conducted the evaluation of DDT as indoor residual spraying (IRS) in the control of Kala-Azar with the objective to assess the susceptibility status of *P. argentipes* to DDT and other commonly used insecticides (Kishore et al.). Limited literature is available on sandfly resistance to DDT in Bihar. Some studies suggest that in many pockets the sandflies have developed resistance against DDT due to its regular use.

This also emphasizes the need for alternative control strategies against the sandfly vectors.

The studies have the susceptibility and resistance of different synthetic insecticides *Phlebotomus* papatasi, another sandfly found along with *P. argentipes* has been reported to be resistant to DDT, Malathion, dieldrin and propoxur (Singh and Bansal, 1996) in different parts of India:

Herbal Control: Alternative for Sandfly Control?

Current efforts to control leishmaniasis are primarily focused on chemotherapy, vector control through the use of chemicals, destruction of rodent burrows and termite moulds, use of impregnated dog collars, environmental manipulation and improvement of housing. Personal protections through the use of lotions and chemical impregnated bed nets are also major tools in vector control (Tonui, 2006). However, these control strategies have been hampered by various factors including rampant spread of drug resistance, high cost of classical anti-leishmanial drugs, lack of suitable vaccines and resistance to the insecticides by vectors. Alternative compounds and especially botanicals are critical sources of ideal control agents because they are safe to most flora and fauna. Control interventions call for a better understanding of the biology and diversity of leishmania parasites, sand flies and the reservoir hosts (Tonui, 2006).

Table 7: Status of Susceptibility and Resistance of Different Synthetic Insecticides in Different parts of India

Vector	*Locality*	*Insecticide*	*Mortality %/ Susceptibility/ Resistance*	*Year*	*Reference*
P. argentipes	Patna (Bihar)	DDT	R/S (86.6-100%)	1990	Mukhopadhyay et al. 8
P. argentipes	Chandauli (Buxar, Bihar)	DDT	R (40%)	1990	
P. argentipes	Mahali (Samastipur, Bihar)	DDT	R (40%)	1990	
P. argentipes	Patna (Bihar)	DDT	R/S (86.6-100%)	1990	
P. argentipes	Bhojpur (Bihar)	DDT	R (40%)	1990	
P. argentipes	Samastipur (Bihar)	DDT	S (100%)	1990	
P. argentipes	Sahebganj (Jharkhand)	DDT	R (82%)	1991	NMEP
P. argentipes	Patepur (Bihar)	DDT	R	1992	WHO 9
P. papatasi	Patepur (Bihar)	DDT	R	1992	
P. argentipes	Vaishali (Bihar)	DDT	R	1992	
P. papatasi	Vaishali (Bihar)	DDT	R	1992	
P. argentipes	Patna (Bihar) Unsprayed	DDT	S (100%)	1993	Kaul et al
P. argentipes	Patna (Bihar) Sprayed	DDT	R (15.4%)	1993	
P. argentipes	Vaishali (Bihar)	DDT	R (2.9%)	1993	

P. argentipes	Varanasi (Uttar Pradesh)	DDT	S (100%)	1994	Thaper et al.
P. argentipes	Hoogly (West Bengal)	DDT	S (100%)	1995	Chandra et al.
P. argentipes	Hoogly (West Bengal)	Malathion	S (100%)	1995	
P. argentipes	Hoogly (West Bengal)	Dieldrin	S (100%)	1995	
P. argentipes	South 24-Paragna (West Bengal)	Malathion	S (100%)	1995	Basak and Tandon
P. argentipes	North 24-Paragana (WB)	DDT	S (100%)	1996	
P. argentipes	South 24-Paragna (WB)	DDT	R (0%)	1996	
Here R = Resistant and S = Susceptible					

Plant-derived products such as azadirachtin from neem (*Azadirachta indica*) have shown potency as insect-growth regulators and are therefore ideal for future use as effective insecticides (Wood, 1990). Crude plant extracts and inorganic larvicides were largely used as natural insecticides before the organic laboratory-synthesized insecticides became available in the 1940s (Balandrin et al., 1985; Raw, 1986; Rozendaal, 1997). Plant extracts such as pyrethrum, nicotine and rotenone were among the first compounds used to control insects of medical and agricultural importance (Grainge and Ahmed, 1988; Coats, 1994). Pyrethrins, a complex of esters extracted from flowers of *Chrysanthemum cinerariefolium* (Compositae), are still used to enhance commercial preparations of household insecticides (Bel et al., 1990). Nicotine extracts from *Nicotiana glauca* and its nicotinoid derivatives are choice molecules for the manufacture of new insecticides.

Rotenone and rotenoids, isoflavanoids found in several genera of tropical leguminosae plants such as Derris (*Papillionaceae*), Antonia (*Loganiaceae*) and Lonchocarpus (*Fabaceae*), were shown to have insecticidal properties against Lutzomyia longipalpis Lutz and Neiva, the vector for *Leishmania chagasi* in Brazil (Luitgards-Moura et al., 2002). Essential lemon oil was found to be 70% protective against sandfly bites (Rojas et al., 1991). A concentration of two percent neem oil mixed in coconut or mustard oil provided 100% protection against *P. argentipes* throughout the night in field conditions (Sharma et al., 1993). Pyrethrin esters have been found to be effective repellents against *P. argentipes* the vector of Indian Kala-Azar (Kishore et al., 2006).

A concentration of 2% neem oil mixed in coconut or mustard oil provided 100% protection against *P. argentipes* throughout the night in field conditions. V.P. Sharma and P.C. Dhiman "Neem Oil as a Sandfly

(Diptera: Psychodidae) Repellent, *J Am Mosq Control Assoc,* 1993; 9: 364-66.) Pyrethrin esters were found to be effective repellents against *P. argentipes*, the vector of Indian kala-azar. K. Kishore et. al. Vector Control in Kala-Azar. *Indian J Med Res,* 2006; 123: 467-72).

Various plants and herbal extracts have been found to be useful in different ways. Some of the plant extracts act as repellents while some have larvicidal effects. Some have also been found to be successful against the adult vectors and still many extracts have also been found to be useful against the parasite *L. donovani* and other similar species.

The repellent action of neem oil has been evaluated against different vector species of malaria in the Mandla District of MP, Ghaziabad District of UP, Hardwar District of Uttarkhand, Kheda District of Gujarat, Panji of Goa and Sonapur of Assam. In these places, various concentrations of neem oil [1 to 4%] was prepared by mixing it with coconut oil or mustard oil and then applied. Two to five ml of neem oil was applied to the exposed body parts of human volunteers and the results were found to be very exciting by Dua et. al. (1995) and Singh et al (1996). Vanishing cream with 5% neem oil has also been prepared in collaboration with Department of Pharmaceuticals, Jamia Hamdard. Results have been seen to reveal that neem cream provides 67 to 100% protection against malaria mosquitoes in different ecological terrains. Neem oil soaked mats in 5% and 10% concentration have been tested as mosquito repellent in a village of Delhi. Results revealed that mean catch per night per person in case of Culex quinquefasiatus remained to be 129.7 with 5% mat and 124.9 with 10% mat as compared to 729.8 in the control under natural conditions (Mittal et. al. 2003).

In the past two decades, various indigenous plants and its extracts in addition to the neem (*Azadirachta indica*) have been tested as mosquito repellent at Malaria Research Centre. Oil of *Cymbopogan martini martini, Cymbopogan citrates* and *Cymbopogan nardus* has been found to provide more than 95% protection against *Culex* and *Anopheles sp.* in whole night landing collection on human baits. Similarly, flowers of *Lantana camara*, extracted in methanol and mixed with coconut oil has been found to provide 94.5% protection against *Aedes sp.* in field conditions. Essential oil extracted by steam distillation of *Mentha piperita* has been found to provide 84.5-100% protection against *Culex quinquefasciatus* and *Anopheles culicifacis* during the whole night landing collection (Sukumar et al., 1991).

Besides repellency effect, various plant products have also been tested for the insecticidal activities against mosquito larvae and adult stages. In addition to the mosquito repellent action, neem oil and other commercial preparation of neem have also been found as potential mosquito larvicide. Neem oil has been found to produce immediate mortality as well as delayed effect by larval growth inhibition. Control of mosquito breeding has been demonstrated in small habitats using indigenous methods of application of neem oil in water and neem oil coated on wooden scraps. Beside neem oil, latex of *Calotropis procera* have been found to produce 100% mortality of larvae of some anopheles species, culex species and *Aedes aegypti* at 1% concentration. Steam distilled oil extracts of *Tagetes errecta* and *Mentha piperita* have been found to produce 100% mortality against mosquito larvae of *An. stephensi*, *Cx. quinquefasciatus* and *Ae. aegypti* at doses lesser than 100 ppm. Crude extract of leaves of *Solanum nigrum* in water has been seen to show larvicidal activity against *An. culicifacies*, *Culex sp.* and *Ae. aegypti* at a dose equivalent to LC90 ranging between 0.18 and 0.21%.

Table 8: Larvicidal Activity of Various Herbal Products Against Vector Mosquitoes

Plant species	*Plant product*	*Species tested*	*References*
Nicotinatobaccum	Nicotin	*Cx. Quinquefasciatus, An. Stephensi, Aedes aegypti*	Cam'bel et al., 1993
Mentha piperita	Essential oil	*Cx. Quinquefasciatus, An. Stephensi, Ae. aegypti*	Ansari et al., 1999
Azadirachta indica	Neem oil	*Cx. quinquefasciatus*	Sharma, 1993
	Neem bark	*An. stephensi*	Mittal et al., 1995
	Neem oil-water	*Cx. quinquefasciatus*	Batra, et al., 1998
	Emulsion	*An. stephensi, Ae. aegypti*	
Tagetus errecta	Steam distilled essential oil	*Cx. quinquefasciatus, Ae. aegypti, An. stephensi*	Pathak et al., 2000
Murraya koengii	Steam distilled essential oil	*Cx. quinquefasciatus, Ae. aegypti, An. stephensi*	Pathak et al., 2000
Solanum nigrum	Leaf extract	*An. Culicifacies, Cx. quinquefasciatus, Ae. aegypti.*	Singh et al., 2001

Table 9: Repellent Activities of Some Plants

Plant species	*Plant product*	*Species tested*	*Percentage (%) protection*
Azadirachta indica	5-40% Neem oil mixed with coconut/mustard oil as topical application	*An. culicifacies*	80-100
		Cx. Quinquefasciatus	61-100
		Ae. Aegypti	85
		Phlebotomus papatasi	97.6
		Phlebotomus argentipes	100
	5% Neem in a cream-based topical application	*Ae. Aegypti*	84
		Ae. Albopictus	78
		Anopheles spp.	93-100
		Culex spp.	89-94
	5-10% Neem oil impregnated on mats (vapours)	*Anopheles spp.*	98
		Cx. Quinquefasciatus	63
	1% Neem oil in kerosene oil (Smoke)	*An culicifacies*	99-100
		Culex spp.	79-81
Cymbopogan spp	Oil as topical application	An. culicifacies	99-100 for 10 hrs
		Cx. Quinquefasciatus	95-97 for 6 hrs
Lantana camara	Methanol + Coconut oil extract	Ae. Albopictus	94 for 2 hrs
		Ae. Aegypti	50 for 4 hrs
Mentha piperta essential oil	Steam distilled	An. annularis	100
		An. culicifacies	92
		Cx. Quinquefasciatus	85

Table 10: List of Plants with Antileishmanial Property

Plants with antileishmanial	*Plant Family*	*Part(s) used*	*Solvent used*	*References activity*
Tridax procumbens	*Asteraceae*	Whole plant	Methanol	Sánchez et al., 2007; Zelmyet al., 2009.
Urechites andrieuxii	*Apocynaceae*	Leaves and roots	Methanol	Pulido and Serralta, 1993; Argüeta et al., 1994; Manuel et al., 2003
Desmodiumgangeticum	*Fabaceae*	Whole plant	n-butanol	Iwu et al., 1992; Nasib et al., 2005
Pseudelephantopus	*Asteraceae*	Leaves, aerial	Ethanol	Odonneet al., spicatus parts 2011
Himatanthussucuuba	*Apocynaceae*	Stem bark,	Ethanol	Villages et al., 1997; Castillo et al., 2007
Azadirchtaindica	*Meliaceae*	Stem bark	Methanol	Ahmed et al., 1998
Maytenussenegalensis	*Celasteraceae*	Stem bark	Methanol	Ahmed et al., 1998
Pseudocedrelakotscifye Balanitesaegyptiaca	*Meliaceae* *Balanitaceae*	Stem bark Seeds, stem bark	Methanol Methanol	Ahmed et al., 1998 Ahmed et al., 1998
Eucalyptus globulus	*Myrtaceae*	Seeds	Methanol	Ahmed et al., 1998

Acanthospermumhispidum	*Asteraceae*	Aerial parts	Dichloromethane	Joanne et al., 2011
Cymbopogoncitratus	*Poaceae*	Leaves	Fresh leaves were steam distilled using Clevenger's apparatus	Santin et al., 2001
Peschieraaustralis	*Apocynaceae*	Stem	Ethanol	Delorenzi et al., 2000
Lantana ukambensis	*Verbenaceae*	Stem, leaves	Methanol	Sawadogo et al., 2012
Chondodendrontomentosum	*Menisper-*	Bark and leaves	Ethanol	González-Coloma
	maceae			et al., 2011
Cedrelaodorata L	*Meliaceae*	Bark	Chloroform,	González-Coloma hexane e t al., 2011
Pentacaliadesiderabilis	*Asteraceae*	Leaves	Methanol	Thiago et al., 2012
Drimysbrasiliensis Miers	*Winteraceae*	Stem barks	Hexane	Daniela et al., 2011
Polyalthialongifolia	*Annonaceae,*	Leaves	Ethanol	Pragya et al., 2010
Valerianawallichii	*Valerianaceae*	Roots	Chloroform, methanol	Ghosh et al., 2011

Literature review shows that more studies need to be carried out on the Indian species as they may show different effects and even the same species might show some different results due to varying climatic conditions. There are more plants that need to be tested against sandflies depending upon their availability which have shown insecticidal effect on other insects. Different extraction methods may be employed for different plant parts for testing the efficacy on sandflies because the effect depends on method of extraction. The plant extracts obtained from different methods can be evaluated for cost effectiveness and self life properties. The anti-leishmanial activity of various plants as shown in Table 10 also suggests that these plants can be used to treat leishmaniasis. It should however be emphasized that reported results in this work have shown that the level of activity of a particular plant depends largely on the solvent used for extraction and to some extent the part of the plant used.

To conclude, it may be assumed that in nature there remain many plants whose extracts have good deal of insecticidal properties against the mosquitoes and other dipterans. Some plant extracts might be applied on sandflies for their control as insecticides and repellents. As DDT presently used for spray in Kala-Azar control programme has ecological hazards linked to long-term biomagnifications, alternatives like herbal control which is supposed to be eco-friendly might be a good alternative for the control of kala-azar. However, the cost-effectiveness of these herbal products as well as its residual effect needs to be analysed further to be used on large scale. Research institutions may play a pivotal role in this case.

Steps and Strategies towards Elimination of Kala-Azar

In India, first step in the direction of decreased incidence of Kala-Azar was introduction of residual insecticide spray under National Malaria Control Programme in the year 1953. It led to significant reduction in the cases of Kala-Azar. In Bangladesh Kala-Azar virtually disappeared during the 'Malaria Eradication Programme (1961-1970). In India centrally sponsored Kala-Azar Control Programme was launched in endemic areas in the year 1950. The programme merged with National Rural Health Mission in the year 2005 under the name of National Vector Borne Disease Control Programme (NVBDCP). Kala-Azar is one of the six entities under NVBDCP in India. Government of India in 2002 National Health Policy had set a goal to eliminate Kala-Azar by year 2010, which could not be attained. Presently the Tripartite MoU aims towards reducing the annual incidence of Kala-Azar and post Kala-Azar dermal Leishmaniasis (PKDL) to less than one per 10000 population at the district (or sub-district) level by the end of the year 2015.

As per current situation, uncertainty prevails in achieving this target. Kala-Azar is among the six entities under portfolio of 'Programme for Research Training in Tropical Diseases' (TDR) under World Health Organization. Since its foundation in the year 1975, TDR led five major elimination campaigns for Kala-Azar in South-East Asia.

In 2005, the three countries agreed to initiate a *VL* elimination programme with high level political commitment and the target of reducing annual *VL* incidence to 1/10,000 population by 2015. Favouring factors for Kala-Azar Elimination are: Human beings as the only reservoir host; *Phlebotomus* argentipes the only vector in the region; *VL* focalized in 109 districts in three countries; the disease being easy to diagnose even in field settings through recently developed rK39 dipstick test and can be treated completely with effective drugs.

The five pillars of the *VL* elimination strategy identified so far are:

(i) Providing access to early diagnosis and treatment;
(ii) Strengthening disease and vector surveillance;
(iii) Integrated vector management;
(iv) Social mobilization and networking; and
(v) Operational research.

Kala-Azar Elimination is Planned in Four Phases in South-East Asia

Preparatory phase of two years started in the year 2005 followed by attack phase of five years. Year 2012 marks the start of consolidation phase for next three years followed by maintenance phase of at least two to three years. Signing of tripartite MoU by three countries commences the beginning of preparatory phase. Main activities during this phase were piloting of total spraying operation, establishment of diagnosis and treatment facilities in endemic countries, monitoring and planning. It is followed by the attack phase.

The main activities during this phase included the indoor residual spraying in endemic areas, integrated vector management, early diagnosis and treatment, case detection, and vector surveillance, community mobilization, external country evaluation and building research capacity. Presently, the consolidation phase has started for the next three years. It is aimed to do active surveillance until no increase in the incidence rate of Kala-Azar occurs at the district and sub-district levels in endemic countries. Total coverage spraying is modified to limit indoor residual spraying in endemic areas. This will be followed by maintenance phase intending to do surveillance against reintroduction of Kala-Azar until Kala-Azar is no longer a public health problem. This will be verified by an international review commission followed by certification of the elimination status.

Major strategies of WHO for elimination of Kala-Azar are effective disease surveillance, early diagnosis and treatment, effective vector control, social mobilization of the population at risk, and clinical and operational research. India under NVBDCP is sharing the strategies of effective vector control, like early diagnosis and treatment, Information education communication and capacity building.

Kala-Azar elimination initiative in India under NVBDCP includes patient coding scheme and monthly Kala-Azar reporting format. The coding would be arranged in the order of Country code, state code, district code, PHC code, sub-centre or NGO code and patient code. Patient coding scheme will make it possible to track all the patients up to the village level. Besides this will overcome the double counting of Kala-Azar cases. The coding scheme is still in preparatory phase. The case definition for suspecting Kala-Azar is history of fever of more than two weeks not responding to antibiotics and anti-malarials. The disease usually presents along with splenomegaly, anaemia and progressive weight loss. This is supplemented by laboratory test mainly direct agglutination, rk39 ipstick and ELISA. Nevertheless, all these tests are IgG based which is relatively long lasting. Confirmatory test is the demonstration of parasite in bone marrow, spleen, lymph node aspiration or in the culture medium.

For almost six decades pentavalent antimonials were used for treatment of Kala-Azar until drug resistance emerged in 1970. Newer drugs that are effective and long lasting are Miltefosine and Amphotericin B. Kala-Azar has more than 80 percent mortality if not treated. Subsequently, early diagnosis and treatment is extremely valuable to reduce case fatality. In India, the mainstay of vector control is through indoor residual spraying (IRS) of DDT up to six feet height from the ground done biannually.

IRS has nearly eliminated Kala-Azar from north-eastern states of Assam, Meghalaya and Tripura. IRS is conducted in all villages which reported Kala-Azar cases in the past five years or during the year of spraying and in villages, which are free of Kala-Azar, but are on search for cases of Kala-Azar. In Bangladesh and Nepal, DDT is not recommended under the national policy. Another available option is the use of Pyrethroid. IRS must be carried out within a radius of one kilometre of water bodies harbouring the vector. In addition to Kala-Azar medicines and insecticides, cash assistance is also being provided to endemic states since December 2003 to facilitate effective strategy implementation.

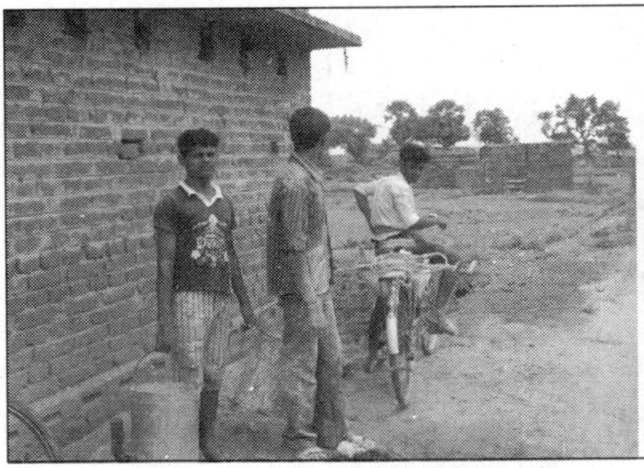

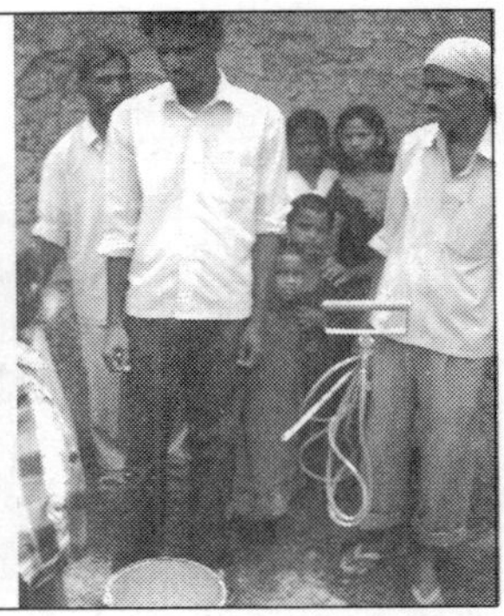

Fig. 22. Fig. 23. Squad members ready for DDT spray

Fig. 24. PIC: complete and patchy

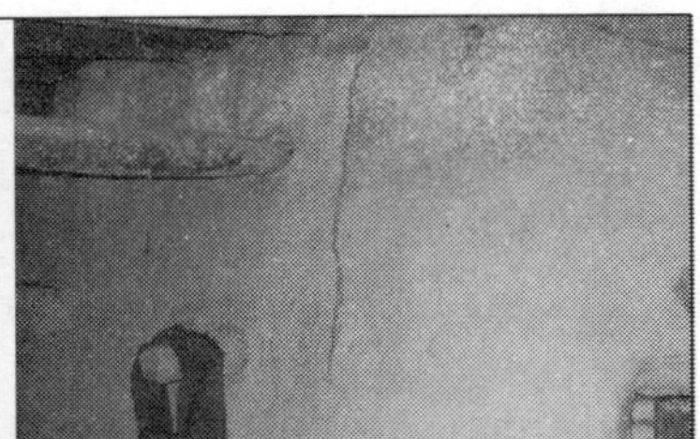

Fig. 25. Spray quality satisfactory spray

For success of elimination, social mobilization is vital. It is required for the success of early diagnosis and treatment, for promoting treatment seeking supporting indoor residual spraying and reducing human vector contact. The NVBDCP is exercising information education and communication system for effective behavioural change communication. More clinical research is required to develop new drugs and diagnostics. New drugs will be required as Amphotericin B. is an injectable preparation whose compliance is poorer as compared to a newer oral preparation and also in India the drug Miltefosine is not freely available.

Treatment

The treatment options for *VL* are limited and far from satisfactory. Pentavalent antimonials (sodium stibogluconate; SbV) and Amp B. have been the two drugs with proven efficacy for treatment of *VL*. Both the drugs are given parenterally and are potentially toxic. Paromomycin, an aminoglycoside antibiotic, is currently undergoing Phase-III clinical trial. Recently, for the first time an oral antileishmanial drug "Miltefosine" has proved effective in treating Indian *VL* and has been registered for treatment of *VL*. Miltefosine has been rolled out in 16 highly endemic districts of Bihar.

Indoor Residual Spray

Indoor residual spraying is most important intervention in achieving the interruption of transmission of diseases transmitted by Phlebotomine sandflies. In 1950s, anti-malaria spraying under the National Malaria Control Programme (NMCP), and National Malaria Eradication Programme (1958) brought about a virtual cessation of Kala-Azar transmission in India. Indoor residual spraying has virtually eliminated Kala-Azar from north-eastern states of Assam, Meghalaya and Tripura and smaller foci in Odissa and Tamil Nadu.

The target of Kala-Azar elimination programme was the interruption of Kala-Azar transmission by the year

2008. Thus, it is imperative that all Kala-Azar villages, whether affected now or in the past, are treated with insecticide sprays. The selection of villages for the spray programme is done by the government as under:

- All villages within a PHC which reported Kala-Azar cases in the past five years.
- All villages which reported cases during the year of spraying.
- Villages which are free of Kala-Azar, but on search are found to contain cases conforming to the Kala-Azar case definition.

The dosage of DDT application is the same as that for anti-malarial spraying, i.e. 1 g/m^2 of the wall surface. The inside walls of huts and cattle shed are to be treated with the insecticide. Spraying is to be restricted to the 6 feet of the wall surface. Cattle sheds and Kala-Azar positive and suspected houses are to be treated on priority.

Spraying is usually started to coincide with the build-up of vector populations and before onset of Kala-Azar transmission. The transmission season of Kala-Azar in India is from June to October. The build-up in population of vector *P. argentipes* starts in March.

The effectiveness of DDT deposits lasts for about 10 weeks. Thus, two rounds of spraying to control *P. argentipes* population are undertaken first in February/March and second in June/July. Two rounds of spray are given for DDT to provide protection during the entire transmission season.

Evaluation of Elimination Technique Adopted in Bihar

The current Kala-Azar Elimination Programme needs to get strengthened by adopting newer strategies. The evidence-based policy should be designed that motivate the implementation of the programmes. Moreover the cost effective policies to controls *VL* will have to include many activities that involve public awareness and modifying personal behaviour.

The five pillars of *VL* elimination strategies identified are: early diagnosis and complete treatment: integrated vector management and vector surveillance, effective disease surveillance through passive and active case detection, social mobilization and building partnerships and clinical & operational research which need to be re-enforced to ensure effective implementation.

Strategies for Surveillance

Government agencies in India collect date via passive case detection (Dejesus, 1999) which grossly underestimates the number of cases. Most cases are diagnosed but not reported by private medical practitioners. Private doctors are not required to report cases to the state health system. The social and cultural stigma linked to *VL* and high prevalence among the poor results in a more percentage of individuals failing to seek treatment at public health facilities (Ranjan et al., 2005). Hence, it is not possible to obtain directly reliable estimated of *VL* incidence using the surveillance system in place.

Under-reporting is one of the main constraints towards the elimination. ASHAs, being the interface between community and health staff, should be utilized and motivated towards active case detection. There should be orientations of ASHA, before each IRS possibly in the months of January and April since these months correspond to those when IRS operations preparation begins. The subsequent months (February and May) should be utilized to inform community regarding the sprays and the necessity of their co-operation for effective surveillance.

In addition, Active Case Detection should be done at least two times in a year in the months of June and

October (at the start and end of the Kala-Azar Transmission Period) similarily as pulse polio rounds. Current incentive for ASHAs (₹ 50 per case for case detection and ₹ 150 for treatment completion) for Kala-Azar should be raised in order to motivate them for active case detection. In Bihar, active case detection is occurring in the camp mode replacing Kala-Azar fortnight, once in a month targeting four villages.

However, this should be done on a wide scale like in polio rounds. IEC/BCC strategies should be employed on a large scale to aggressively search for suspected cases as well as before the IRS. The state has rolled out a national programme, Integrated Disease Surveillance Project (IDSP) to capture morbidity rate of 22 infectious diseases including Kala-Azar as state specific disease under the programme. The programme has some constraints like lack of motivation of private sector to provide information to government system, lack of sufficient manpower in the absence of which assignment of task to a specific person that can bring report from private facilities or practitioners becomes difficult. This is further afflicted with the lack of incentives provided to them with respect to distance they have to cover between private facility and the place where they are supposed to report. Mobility support is also one of the challenges for the health workers which need proper attention.

Entomological surveillance in the state has been weak. The state has initiated a study on monthly vector density to generate Early Warning Signals of impending outbreaks. Study on insecticide susceptibility shows status of vector-borne consultants in endemic districts who can do this surveillance on regular basis. Date sharing between various research institutions in the state and state programme officer needs to be strengthened. Involvement of academic institution can also prove valuable support to the programme.

Community Participation in Kala-Azar Elimination

Since community plays a pivot role towards success of any health programme, community should be motivated towards increasing passive surveillance and support in the Indoor Residual Spray. Efforts should be made to include one of the members from the targeted village to be included in Indoor Residual Sprays for quality improvement of spray. Spray monitoring should be done by the community.

Treatment Procedure: Mitefosine should be rolled out in all the districts and since clinical half-life of mitefosine is long (170 hours) and there is a possibility of resistance to the same, DOTS guidelines should be prepared and introduced. DOTS providers should be identified and additional incentives should be provided to them for DOTS. A referral system should be established for Kala-Azar patients. Patients should be given some incentives for travel to PHC or referral or higher centres for better treatment.

PKDL and HIV/TB co-infection with Kala-Azar Cases: Active surveillance with special efforts to find PKDL cases should be intensified. There should be establishment of a Regional Health Centre equipped to deal with PKDL, HIV and TB co-infected and for other unresponsive cases. A specialist should be made available to treat all such cases. Special incentives should be provided to PKDL cases treated completely. There should be the provision for skin biospy at the district hospitals in all the districts of Bihar.

Nutrition

Rapidly developing anaemia is one of the symptoms in Kala-Azar and since this develops rapidly and accounts for malnutrition, treatment of anaemia should be included along with medications. A special diet with good nutritious value and fortified with iron should be developed and provided to Kala-Azar patients.

Strategies of Vector Control

In addition to chemical control using IRS, vector control should be supplemented by other hygiene measures. LLINs are effective against sandfly. Houses with cracks and crevices should be filled with mud or lime before the spray. Cow-dung being one of the important sources of sandfly breeding is managed in different ways. Before the night, cow-dung should be collected and dried on the roof or some place more than six feet high.

One of the remarkable traditions in Bihar is sleeping in the cattle-shed in order to prevent stealing of cattle and this can be a site of sandfly bite. There should be a recommendation of developing a (Mechan) wooden block which should be installed at a height of six feet for sleeping and mandate of using Long Lasting Insecticide Nests (LLINs) for any person sleeping in cattle-shed. Some studies show resistance of sand flies to DDT in some areas of Bihar. There should be continuous operational research to find out resistance to DDT in area with high prevalence and provision of using alternate insecticides.

Need of Clinical and Operational Research

There should be consistent clinical and operational research towards finding out compliance to the drugs and implementation of different strategies and their effects. Entomological studies should be regularly carried out finding out newer advances for sandfly control.

Environmental Modifications

Since Kala-Azar affects the poorest segments of the society; there should be the provision of proper housing in highly-endemic Kala-Azar prone areas. Govt. of India has taken initiatives in the form of construction of *Pucca* houses to Mushahar community and ₹ 12.03 crores have already been released under Indira Vikas Yojana to the State of Bihar.

Inter- and Intra-sectoral Convergence

A Kala-Azar Task Force should be made functional. The members of this task force should include members from both health and non health sectors. This would help in sensitizing the community from all spheres regarding Kala-Azar prevention, treatment and elimination.

Future Planning for Kala-Azar Elimination

To combat the problem of treatment failure in Kala-Azar and to reduce the length of therapy, combination of at least two effective anti-leishmanial agents needs to be assessed. Regular availability of drugs around the year, good-quality drugs, less waiting time at clinics, easily approachable doctors with good communication skills and flexible clinic hours may ensure greater compliance. Over the counter, sale of anti-leishmanial drugs should be restricted. This could be a major step towards preventing the emergence of resistance against anti-leishmanials. Reporting of cases of PKDL should be an integral part of the surveillance and monitoring system. Early identification can be improved by counselling Kala-Azar patients on the risks and the signs of PKDL during their treatment. Improved detection of PKDL cases by health workers would be useful. The PCR should be promoted for the diagnosis of PKDL. Supervised treatment could be a way for improving treatment compliance by patients.

Environmental management for vector control (EVM) and integrated vector management (IVM) should be emphasized more. The role of newer methods like long-lasting insecticide-treated nets and plastering household walls need to be explored for effective vector management. Community cooperation is to be gained for indoor residual spraying. A vaccine against leishmaniasis for general human use is still under trial. Presence of an effective vaccine is one of the pillars for achieving elimination. One major factor for a vaccine not being in use is the lack of perception of a market for human leishmaniasis vaccines.

Moreover, leishmaniasis is a regional problem and not global one. Endemic country of SEAR needs to conduct active case detection to estimate the correct burden of disease. This could include house-to-house surveillance also known as blanket screening, the index case approach using snowballing, a camped base approach or an incentive-based approach.

Nearly 50% of the problem of Kala-Azar is in the districts located on international borders. The porous border between India and Nepal accentuates the problem through population movements, including migration. Regular exchange of information at the local level across borders, institutional networking for capacity development and use of similar protocols for diagnosis and treatment and synchronization of prevention efforts can contribute significantly to the elimination efforts.

A number of strategies and tools exist to improve global health that can be applied to Kala-Azar. Improved information systems need to be constructed so that the epidemiology, transmission and burden of Kala-Azar and PKDL are accurately assessed. Effective behavioural change communication is needed to sensitize the people. Various forms of local advertisement like street plays, health talks, hoardings and other methods, along with electronic media will prove to be a powerful tool for this. Public-private partnership and involvement of NGOs need to be strengthened in order to provide better services to Kala-Azar patients. Public-private partnership is essential to boost funding and support. Political commitment and development of accountability is the need of the hour. Though three endemic countries have three more years to achieve the set targets, we are still far from our targets.

Recent Development

Union Government has vowed to criminate Kala-Azar from Bihar and other parts of the country by 2015. For this, the Ministry will take a slew of steps including providing Ambisome injection that cures the disease with a single shot. Bihar, incidentally, accounts for 80% Kala-Azar cases in the world, with 33 districts of the state affected by the disease. Ambisome injection, which costs $18 each, will be funded by WHO and other agencies to the Government of India. Ambisome, experts say, will prove to be a milestone because of its 98% efficacy. In the first phase, the new treatment protocol will be introduced in Vaishali, Saran, Sitamarhi, East Champaran and Saharsa districts.

The national road map for tackling the disease was unveiled by the minister at a meeting held with the health officials of four states – Bihar, West Bengal, Jharkhand and Uttar Pradesh. To stress upon the prevention component, the Health Ministry has decided to replace DDT with Synthetic Pyrethroid for the purpose of fogging that eliminates sandfly, which spreads Kala-Azar through its bite. DDT was not effective in a few districts as sandfly had developed resistance to it. For the first time, incentives have been introduced in the programme against kala-azar. An ASHA worker will be given ₹ 300 each for identifying a Kala-Azar patient and ₹ 100 for ensuring community support during spraying. Even the patient being treated in hospital will be given ₹ 500 as "compensation of daily wage for the time he has spent in the hospital during treatment".

The Union and State Governments have also decided on time-bound initiatives for checking Kala-Azar in 33 districts of Bihar. For search of Kala-Azar patients in blocks and villages, a special four-day survey will be launched from September 5 at Araria, Purnia, Muzaffarpur, Vaishali, Saran, East Champaran, Gopalganj, Sharasa, Samastipur and Sitamarhi districts.

The survey in rest of the districts will be completed by December. The training of health officials concerned in the districts on the new treatment protocol will take place from September 5 to September 10. While the respective DMs will monitor the plan at block and district level, the state-level monitoring will be done by the Chief Minister himself.

Incidentally, Kala-Azar mostly occurs among the poorest of poor living in mud houses where sandfly breeds. Effective spraying is the key to elimination of the disease. The Health Ministry has also asked the State Government to build *pucca* houses for the poor because sandfly mostly breeds in mud houses.

Strategy for Tackling the Problem

This has five components:

(i) Indoor residual spray by DDT: It is to break the human-vector-human transmission. This is programmed for blanket spray twice a year in all villages where a case has been reported in the last three years. This is to be done in Feb-March when the flies are said to be most active and in June July (this is what WHO says, the programme suggested May June – it is not clear why there is a different view – maybe because it would be impractical in flood affected areas of North Bihar in July) which is said to be their breeding season. Perhaps it the same period for Jharkhand too.

(ii) Early detection: However, at present detection is largely passive in nature which means that a patient having symptoms and fever for more than 15 days will seek medical care. Other signs are enlarged spleen and liver, which people may not be able to easily perceive on their own. The problem is that initial symptoms mimic many other conditions – non-specific viral fever, enteric fever and malaria. Rapid diagnostic tests are being used. Bihar has planned to have seven active case detection camps in each PHC in a year, though the advice is quarterly. There should be a revision. Camps should be many more in high risk PHCs perhaps supplemented by house-to-house search. We were told that RMRI has concluded that house to house search is too resource intensive. We are not talking of an outside campaign but a much simpler approach using the personnel available. There also need to be five guidelines for this purpose. It has to be done at level of ASHA's and supported by the consultant and KTS.

(iii) Curing the detected patients: Treatment regimen is currently use of oral drug Miltefosine. Drug administration is on DOT basis. Treatment compliance remains an issue because it lasts for 28 days. Combination treatment therapy with Miltefosine + Paromomycine (10 days treatment) is being tried in seven identified districts. Single day Ambisome (1 day treatment) is being tried out at the MSF wards at District Hospital in hajipur. These drugs are provided by MSF.

(iv) IEC: In order to ensure the above two, IEC is carried out. However, its effectiveness as currently conducted is questionable.

(v) Capacity building of staff: This appears to be a routine but continuous activity. ASHAs' capacities certainly need upgradation. The real problem is the vacancies and the ability to deliver.

□

8
Constraints in Kala-Azar Elimination

Kala-Azar Elimination Programme

In 2005, *VL* elimination programme was initiated with high-level political commitment and the target of reducing annual *VL* incidence to 1/10,000 population by 2015.

Favouring factors are: human beings the only reservoir host; *Phlebotomus argentipes* the only vector in the region; *VL* focalized in 109 districts in three countries; the disease easy to diagnose even in field settings through recently developed rK39 dipstick test and can be treated completely with effective drugs.

The five pillars of the *VL* elimination strategy identified so far are:

(i) providing access to early diagnosis and treatment;
(ii) strengthening disease and vector surveillance;
(iii) integrated vector management;
(iv) social mobilization and networking; and
(v) operational research.

Key Programme Constraints

(a) Technical:

- Active Case Search is done only fortnightly and is labour-intensive. Generally the yield of cases are very low.

- Continued dependence on Napierís Aldehyde test for diagnosis of Kala-Azar except in pilot districts.
- Emerging trend of poor response to first line drug Sodium Stibo Gluconate (SSG) in North Bihar which is also toxic when the prescribed regime for 28 days treatment is strictly followed.
- Despite clear guidelines from GoI, indiscriminate use of medicines and incomplete treatment are common among both public and private sector health service providers.
- Treatment protocols are not followed properly.
- Treatment cards recommended for use under programme often are not filled adequately.
- Detection of Post Kala-Azar Dermal Leishmaniasiss (PKDL) and its treatment is not satisfactory. The treatment is prolonged and patients have no motivation to follow the treatment since they do not suffer any ill-health except for the skin problems.
- Coverage and quality of IRS is unsatisfactory.
- Emergence of HIV-Kala-Azar and TB-Kala-Azar co-infections.

(b) Operational

- Political commitment exists but insufficient monitoring of control interventions and resource utilization; variable absorption capacity of states in relation to utilization of funds/commodities.
- A large number of patients receive treatment through private sector which does not report these cases and treatment outcomes to the government. Though Kala-Azar is included under the notifiable diseases in Bihar, enforcement needs to be addressed effectively.

- A large number of patients do not complete the recommended 28 days treatment because of poverty, side effects of medicine and weak supervision by the health-care providers.
- Limited social mobilization due to inadequate BCC efforts with low resource allocation.

(c) Management

- Non-receipt of funds by the districts/PHCs due to administrative delays or non-release of funds by states.
- Non-submission of SOEs and UCs by the states thus hampering release of funds by the GoI.

Challenges Towards Kala-Azar Elimination

Based on the information given above, we come across the following challenges to the programme:

1. Under-reporting
2. Weak surveillance including that for PKDL
3. No or poor quality monitoring of IRS
4. Treatment non-compliance
5. Detection and treatment of PKDL cases are challenging
6. Private sector not reporting the cases.
7. Community resistance to IRS.

The key indicators of Kala-Azar elimination are case detection rate, treatment completion rate, coverage rate for vector control and social mobilization. The burden of Kala-Azar is grossly underestimated by the health systems in the Indian sub-continent due to over-reliability on passive surveillance. Though Kala-Azar patients ultimately report to health centres and hospitals, diagnosis is often missed in the early stages of infection and delayed due to lack of diagnostic facilities at peripheral levels of the health system with a consequent delay in treatment and sustaining the human reservoir.

Besides this, unavailability of non-invasive rapid diagnostic test aggravates the delay in the diagnosis.

Many Kala-Azar cases go undiagnosed in a web of unqualified medical practitioners which further add to considerable delay in diagnosis and treatment. Patients who are going to private sector for treatment usually stop in between due to high cost, leading to prolonged transmission.

Strategies are to improve reporting by strengthening diagnosis and treatment besides involving the private sector. To give pace to the elimination, Kala-Azar could be addressed as notifiable disease. This will not only help to estimate the true burden of Kala-Azar but also hasten the treatment of patients identified with better monitoring. There is a wide gap in training and support of staff with technical and management expertise. As prevention and control activities for Kala-Azar are increasing in India, there is a need to strengthen the health system.

The Poly-parasitism and co-infections are major emerging problems in the world of Kala-Azar. In recent years, the threat of HIV and Kala-Azar co-infection is amplifying. To date, co-infection with leishmaniasis and HIV has reached 35 countries. The risk of developing Kala-Azar in endemic areas is about 100 to 1000 times higher in individuals infected with HIV. HIV infection also impairs treatment response and increases the likelihood of recurrence. If HIV epidemic spreads to the general population where Kala-Azar is endemic, it may have disastrous consequences.

Resistance was reported for DDT indoor residual spraying and uses of insecticide treated nets are inconclusive, so there is a need to assess alternative vector control methods. Governmental indoor residual spraying was not in operation in Bangladesh until 2010 and sub-optimum in India and Nepal during the attack phase. A research strategy is required to develop new methods for vector control considering air and water pollution, deforestation, habitat fragmentation, ecological disruption and changing agricultural practices, which have an impact on the incidence, prevalence and spread of infectious diseases.

Post Kala-Azar Dermal Leishmaniasis (PKDL) patients have probably epidemiological importance in Kala-Azar transmission as the lesions can harbour a large amount of leishmania parasites, and as such could constitute a reservoir in the community capable of triggering a new epidemic. As PKDL causes little or no clinical discomfort, and PKDL treatment with intramuscular SSG injections is long (3-4 months), painful and cumbersome, few patients seek treatment.

A generic Miltefosine pharmaceutical product emerged in Bangladesh for the treatment of *Visceral leishmaniasis* and is used in the national elimination programme. Poor-quality drugs for the treatment of this fatal neglected tropical disease are not only life-threatening but also have a devastating impact on public health and elimination programme targeting this disease. Kala-Azar patients belong to the poorest quintile of the population, which make them highly dependent for drug provision by national elimination programme. These extremely vulnerable patients deserve to be protected by national or regional drug regulators who should take responsibility by implementing the necessary precautions to prevent poor-quality drugs. Shortage and supply delays of Kala-Azar drugs, unavailability of diagnostics at the health centre level often contributes to the community's poor public perception of the public health systems and as consequent low community participation in Kala-Azar control programme activities. Production of medicines for neglected tropical diseases ought to become attractive to manufacturers of generic drugs.

Kala-Azar may not affect the national economy or the national GDP, but it devastates the families affected. This is because the poorest of the poor who are maximally affected by the disease sink deeper into poverty following an attack of Kala-Azar. The strategy for elimination of Kala-Azar should focus inter-sectoral coordination aimed at improving the socio-economic status of the poorest of the poor in the community. Kala-Azar leads to a loss of about four lakhs DAILYs every year in Nepal amounting to a loss of approximately US$ 140 million annually. The evidence-based policy needs to be developed to make Programme more cost-effective.

Elimination of Kala-Azar in member countries of the WHO South-East Asia Region is relevant for achieving the Millennium Development Goals (MDGs) by alleviating poverty. Policies to control Kala-Azar will have to include many activities that involve public awareness and modifying behaviour. Planning of prevention and control measures for Kala-Azar should take into account the possible effects of migrants and moving population. The allocated budget per person per annum for risk population by national programme for Bangladesh, India and Nepal as estimated are around 0.2, 0.4 and 0.3 US$ for Bangladesh, India and Nepal, respectively. Supports from international agencies and non-governmental organizations need to be achieved to overcome the economic constrains.

Governance Issues

The various issues raised here suggest that the main problem is of governance and accountability at the state level and below. WHO prepared a road map with definite action points and timelines in 2013 at the instance of the State. It is unfortunate that nothing has happened. In fact, preparations have worsened, as far as the actions from the state are concerned. We were told that Jharkhand has prepared a good road map. Unless there is commitment, elimination, and later prevention of recurrence, it will not happen or will get delayed. Problems and solutions are well known. The following issues are important, which require to be addressed urgently:

i. A public declaration from the political executive that every effort will be made to eliminate Kala-Azar by 2015.

ii. Secretary Health and ED, NRHM in Govt. of India to give some portion of their time to Kala-Azar and personally monitor critical issues. Visits to the states are made.

iii. The Collector of the District must be made in charge of this programme since we are now in elimination mode. (JMM has recommended CMO to be in charge – he already is, with little impact, unfortunately.)

iv. All vacancies to be filled up in the next six months. This applies to KTS and Kala-Azar Consultants. It also requires that there be a proper officer in charge of the programme at State level and in at least the critical KA districts (maybe 7-8 – he may have additional charge of a smaller district).

v. Revisions be immediately made in the salaries of some staff bringing parity wherever required with other programmes, and also provision of mobility (including costs of insurance and service, etc. – motorcycles are not insured), and perhaps some mobile charges.

vi. In a camp mode, in the next two months, all expenditure statements are compiled, collected and received and all arrear payments made. And system is set up to ensure this to be done on a monthly basis henceforth.

vii. Spatial analysis be done immediately within the next three months, both for cluster of villages within blocks and for households within the endemic villages.

viii. Start focal spray immediately keeping elections in mind. This spray will be where cases have been found in the last two years. Plan as per strategy suggested.

ix. ASHA's role and capacity be immediately addressed. Active case detection strategies should be implemented.

x. WHO should provide state level consultants, as suggested, for a period of three years. An advisory group should also be set up. It could visit quarterly.

xi. Ensure drug procurement at central level without delay.

A very brief JMM note after the mission suggests the following: "to achieve elimination by 2015, programme needs serious acceleration of evidence-based quality operations at all levels. A polio type approach might be considered by both Central and involved States where high level advocacy should also be made to ensure the stewardship and ownership role of State Government." It adds "a periodic external assessment of the progress of Kala-Azar elimination programme has to be undertaken".

They have recommended external assessment of spray operations; development of cost effectiveness in spray; spatial analysis; 'cemented' housing; active case detection; procure best RDT kits, etc.

□

9

Involvement of Developmental Partners

The developmental partners play very crucial role in containing Kala-Azar disease, as the present efforts are more from developmental partners than from the government sectors. The roles of key developmental partners are as under:

1. World Health Partners (WHP)

The organization works on detection and treatment of four key diseases – TB, Kala-Azar, and childhood diarrhoea and childhood pneumonia. This is a five year project 2011-16, funded by Bill and Melinda Gates Foundation. The project implementation began in March 2011. They are currently working in 13 districts in phase I and shall cover another 12 districts in phase II. They work on the Social Franchise Model and Engage (Sky Care providers) private and rural medical practitioners involving quacks and Ayurvedic specialists as well. They are mainly using RMPs and include the training for the diagnostic symptoms, diagnosis – both by clinical and laboratory techniques. The Sky Care providers are given training on the diagnosis of Kala-Azar using rk39 and refer the positive patients to the nearby govt. facilities. The serious patients or those requiring the in-patient treatment are referred to the nearby franchise clinic. They have developed the SKY telemedicine centre and a central medical laboratory at Patna and Delhi.

The telemedicine centres cover an area of 8-10 RMPs. The telemedicine centre (Sky Health Centre) provides the facilities for the remote diagnosis and audio-visual communications between the patients and qualified medical practitioners at Central Medical Facility. Each Sky Health Centre is run by a person of the same village who should be at least matriculate. For establishing telemedicine centre, each entrepreneur is paid an assistance of ₹ 30,000 that includes the space, computer and Internet facilities. No incentive is paid to the Sky Care providers for referring the patients to the govt. facilities (however they plan to get some incentives in the near future and efforts are going on in that direction). RK39 for Kala-Azar has been provided from the Govt. and for telemedicine centres, have been developed by WHP. Sky Care providers can directly call any specialist at central medical laboratory for any suspected case and take their expert opinion. Moreover he may refer the patient to telemedicine centre where the patient can have a face-to-face chat with the specialist and get the expert opinion. In each district they have district programme officer taking care of the telemedicine and Sky Care providers.

In each district they have one District Programme Coordinator and two field officers and one monitoring officer. District programme coordinator is responsible for the whole operations in the district. Field officers are involved in identification of providers, liaising with the trainings, and Rk39 kits distribution. Monitoring officers are responsible for the client verification.

Currently, they are receiving rk39 from the govt. and is the only support they have from the govt. They have the training materials for identification of suspects. BCC is under development. Video displaying the use of rk39 for training the Sky Care providers will be available by the end of the December and posters displaying the case identification to be made available at each facility by the end of January. Client based IEC-BCC shall be rolled out in Feb.

2. Medecins Sans Frontieres (MSF)

The organization is working in DH and five PHCs in district Vaishali since July 2007 and has treated around 7000 patients. They have taken a ward at District Hospital, Hajipur and provide diagnosis, treatment to the Kala-Azar patients using ambisome (liposomal amphotericin B.). Community awareness programmes are being undertaken on weekly basis in different areas. IEC staff unit at office go to the block and provide sensitization for Kala-Azar in the community meetings. They provide treatment to all kinds of patients including the PKDL ones. They have their IEC materials and provide training to ASHAs using their field staff. They were buying ambisome with their own funds.

3. Bihar Voluntary Health Association (BVHA)

BVHA (VHAI) signed a MoU with the GoI in April 2011. The project is centrally funded by NVBDCP and supported by World Bank. The project was supposed to start in December, but is delayed due to the unavailability of IEC materials which is currently getting developed by New Concept. BVHA will work in 31 endemic districts and covers 15,000 highly endemic population/district (nearly 20-25 villages/district). The implementation is done by 20 NGO partners. For each district, they will have a district supervisor and two cluster supervisors (population – 75000/each cluster) and one ASHA for each of 1000 population. ASHA and the supervisors shall be trained on Kala-Azar and sprays. For each case, ASHA shall be provided an incentive of ₹ 22 by BVHA in addition to ₹ 50 as per the VBD guidelines.

Activities

1. Active Case search for Kala-Azar suspected cases by ASHA and group of people chosen by district and cluster supervisors.
2. The supervisors shall educate the community regarding the Kala-Azar and sprays which shall be decided by the supervisors themselves.
3. The supervisors shall monitor and ensure that the patient goes to the PHC for treatment and is compliant to the treatment.
4. The supervisors shall motivate the community to use Long Lasting Insecticide Nets (LLIN).

4. Department of International Development-Bihar Technical Assistance and Support Team (DFID-BTAST)

BTAST is a team formed by the Consortium of three consulting firms – Care India, IPE Global (Infrastructure Professional Enterprise) and Options-UK to support a Government of Bihar-DFID collaborate project "Sector Wide Approach to Strengthen Health" (SWASTH). SWASTH is a six-year project beginning from 2010 and works towards bringing out health sector reforms in the department of Health, Nutrition and Water Sanitation. One of the wings of BTAST works towards bringing out facility improvement in Kala-Azar and tuberculosis, with main focus on Kala-Azar. The project has divided all the health facilities from SC to district hospital into three levels – L1, L2 and L3 on the basis of the minimum services they should provide. The purpose of the project is to bring the existing facilities to that level by providing technical support to the government.

5. DNDI (Drugs for Neglected Diseases Initiative)

DNDI in collaboration with MSF is experimenting to provide short regime for Kala-Azar using combination of the existing drugs.

By above information, we see that the developmental partners are working in different ways. This is of paramount importance that all of them work with proper co-ordination despite working on different platforms.

BVHA is mainly focusing on enhancing surveillance in highly endemic villages and is important one. The under reporting of cases is one of the main challenges of Kala-Azar and can be highly augmented based on the fact that the mass population in Bihar is still less educated and poor. However, BVHA's focus is limited to highly-endemic areas in 31 districts endemic for Kala-Azar and there is a need to expand its operations to other left-out areas. MSF is providing treatment which is not different from the services available in the govt. facilities.

Since the treatment of the Kala-Azar patients is long and full, compliance is still a problem. Hence, treating the PKDL cases is one of the challenges and MSF has been very successful in that. World Health Partners (WHP) are also working towards enhancing surveillance and diagnosis through quacks. Working with or taking help of the quacks may not be a long sustainable idea for India. But in the context of Bihar, quacks play a major role as large number of population visits quacks for any ailments. Diagnosis is done using rk39 and other technical equipment.

However, WHP is limited to 25 districts. DFID-BTAST is working towards improving services in the facilities in the whole State of Bihar in a phased manner. Ensuring diagnosis and treatment to 31 endemic districts and providing manpower is also being taken care of by World Bank assisted project. Despite these supports, in order to achieve elimination goal, there is a need to focus on surveillance and monitoring of the quality of indoor residual spray. Since IRS remains the only method for vector control in India; it constitutes a vital component of Kala-Azar elimination.

There is a need for more co-ordinated efforts of the development partners working in this area. Moreover, community participation is one of the components needed for disease elimination. UNICEF has worked on IEC/BCC in polio eradication programme. There is a need for a partner to work on that as well because resistance is common to DDT spray due to community perceiving it as hazardous chemical and it also leaves a residual blackened effect on the walls. Many residents resist spraying of DDT in particular. This is due to a variety of factors including its smell and the stains it leaves on the walls. While the stains on the walls make it easier to check whether the room has been sprayed, it causes some villagers to resist the spraying of their homes or to resurface the wall, which eliminates the residual insecticidal effect.

□

10
Integrated Policy Perspective for Kala-Azar Control

In India, particularly north Bihar (including Araria, Purnea, and Kishanganj) is the endemic zone of this disease in Bihar while the disease's geographical coverage is broad. The disease clusters around areas of drought, famine, and high population density. In Africa, this means a knot of infection centers mostly in Sudan, Kenya, and Somalia. Living conditions here have changed very little since the past century, and the people are not normally very mobile. Parts of the Sudan, in particular the Upper Nile region, are almost totally cut off from the rest of the country, and the people are as tied to the place of their birth as any peasant of Europe's Dark Ages.

Kala-Azar is endemic in 88 countries, particularly in Africa, Latin America, South and Central Asia, the Mediterranean basin and the Middle East with over 200 million people at risk. In the South-East Asian Region, Kala-Azar is prevalent in India, Bangladesh and Nepal and with few foci in Bhutan. It is endemic in 115 districts spread over this four countries, namely India (52), Bangladesh (45), Nepal (12), and Bhutan (6). In India, Kala-Azar cases are concentrated in Bihar, Uttar Pradesh, West Bengal and Jharkhand with over 165.4 million people at risk. In India there is a resurgence of Kala-Azar in last few years, but overall deaths are declining. (Fig. 20)

Epidemiologically, Kala-Azar follows an epidemic cycle resurging almost every 15-20 years. The population at risk is nearly 65 million, 6 million, and 2.5 million in Bangladesh, Nepal and Bhutan, respectively. Regardless of lots of strategy for elimination estimated annual incidence of Kala-Azar cases are varying from 20-25 in India, 5-8 in Nepal and 13-31 in Bangladesh per 10,000 population.

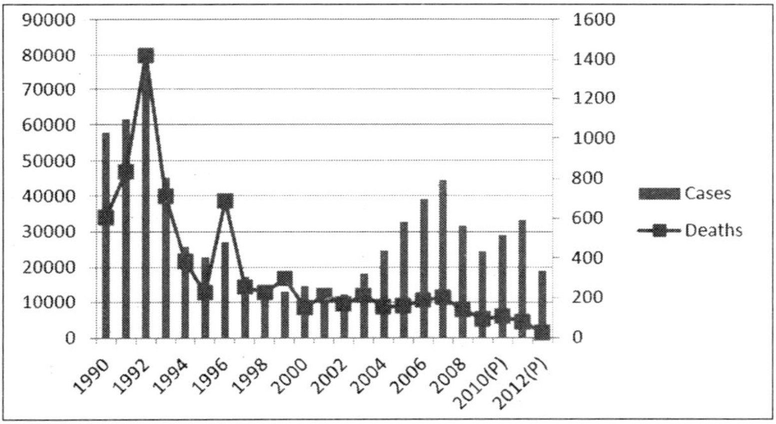

Fig. 20. Trend of cases and death due to Kala-Azar in India (as updated on 08. January, 2013).

World Health Organization: Planning a Pro-active Role

It is rightly mentioned here that the World Health Organization has been playing a laudable role at the international level with a view to ensure the availability of the highest standards of health-care to people all over the world.

The Preamble of the World Health Organization Constitution is as under:

- The enjoyment of the highest standards of health is one of the fundamental rights of every human being without distinction of race, religion, political belief, and economic and social condition.

- The health of all people is fundamental to the attainment of peace and security and is dependent upon the fullest co-operation of individuals and states.
- The achievement of any state in the promotion and protection of health is of value to all.
- Unequal development in different countries in the promotion of health and control of disease, especially communicable disease, is a common danger.
- Healthy development of the child is of basic importance; the ability to live harmoniously in a totally changing environment is essential to such development.
- The extension to all people of the benefits of medical, psychological and related knowledge is essential to the fullest attainment of health.
- Informed opinion and active co-operation on the part of the public are of the utmost importance in the improvement of the health of the people.
- Governments have a responsibility for the health of their people, which can be fulfilled only by the provision of adequate health and social measures.

Article 2 of the same Constitution deals with functions that, directly and indirectly, require the application of legal principles such as:

(i) To act as the directing and co-coordinating authority on international health work;

(ii) To propose "Conventions, Agreements and Regulations", make recommendations with respect to international health matters, and to perform such duties as may be assigned thereby to the Organization and are consistent with its objective; and

(iii) To develop, establish and promote international standards with respect to food, biological, pharmaceutical and consumer products.

Several International Agencies have also Lent Support to Public Participation in Health-care

The World Health Organization in Alma Ata Declaration 1978 states that:

"The people have the right and duty to participate individually and collectively in the planning and implementation of their health-care."

Planning for Kala-Azar Control in India

1. An organized centrally sponsored control programme was launched in endemic areas in 1990-91.
2. Government of India provided Kala-Azar medicines, insecticides and technical support and the State governments implemented the programme through primary health-care system and district/zonal and State malaria control organizations and provided other costs involved in strategy implementation.
3. Programme strategy included:
   - Vector control through IRS with DDT up to 6 feet height from the ground twice annually
   - Early diagnosis and complete treatment
   - Information education communication
   - Capacity building
   - Programme intensified in 1991-92 which led to improved case registration through primary health-care system.
4. Structural Planning

The State Government has made the following structure which has been strengthened by additional assistance from Govt. of India, and further help is coming from other agencies.

I. The programme has been amalgamated with the NRHM. However, there is a State Programme Director for VCDCP including Kala-Azar. In

Bihar, he seems to be dysfunctional. Jharkhand is reportedly better. The point is that a dynamic full time officer needs to be posted, and must remain for the next three years. GoI should have this ensured.

II. At the district level there is supposed to be District Malaria Officer (24 positions for 38 districts). However, for a long time, only one person has been in position – at Muzzaffarpur. Rest of the districts have an officer in additional charge. He cannot, and does not give much time to this programme. How does one provide leadership at the district level at least in the 10-15 critical districts? This problem must be addressed.

III. Bihar was provided with district level consultants under the World Bank project. They continue even after the project has ended under domestic budget. Currently, there are 29 consultants for 33 endemic districts. Jharkhand has only 1 out of 4, and he is supposed to look after malaria too. How can these posts be kept vacant?

IV. Six posts in each district were sanctioned for Kala-Azar treatment supervisor, much like the STS under the RNTCP. 140 out of 186 are reportedly in position in Bihar and 18 out of 24 in Jharkhand. The number six is not related to the need – it is for the district (31×6). Clearly, an urgent redistribution of posts is required among districts, so that the number is more in endemic districts. However, this is somewhat notional as posts even in high endemic districts are not fully filled. Can we afford to keep these important posts vacant? And for months together?

V. There are some malaria inspectors, but it appears their role is peripheral and there is talk that they are usually deputed, quite conveniently for them, for law and order duties.

VI. The normal health-care infrastructure takes care of the rest. Treatment is in the PHCs or district and other hospitals. There are many cases in Sadar hospitals of some districts. There also might be many cases in bigger private hospitals. It needs to be examined why, and from where? ASHAs are supposed to help identify patients with symptoms. However, as mentioned earlier, their capacity needs attention and this task needs to be explicitly given to them so that they get into active mode.

The Medium-term Goals and Vision

Reclaiming public health demanding a system for universal access to appropriate health-care is a right-based framework. We thus find ourselves at a crossroads; health-care can be considered a commodity to be sold, or it can be considered a basic social right. It cannot comfortably be considered both of them at the same time. No doubt, the public health system is in a crisis. Obviously the new national government is forced to adopt certain measures to strengthen public health in order to alleviate the situation. Such measures certainly opens spaces for pro-people civil society and organization policy at various levels.

The Long-term Goals and Vision

For achieving the goals of "Health for All", it requires among other conditions, comprehensive nutritional and food security (linked to livelihood security), universal access to safe drinking water and sanitation, provision of health-related education and information for all, and an equitable, just-gender social milieu free from violence, which should be our larger vision.

The achievement of a strengthened public health system, which is more accountable to ordinary citizens, is a potentially achievable goal to fight for within the existing system.

Similarly, the health movement must lend it strength and voice to movements such as nutritional services and food security, clean drinking water, sanitation and safer environmental and working conditions, which may be achieved to certain extent. Such struggles can lead to some concrete improvement in the situation of the working people, and of various deprived and marginalized sections of society. It can also be one channel for people to assert their strength, by demanding that public institutions work for them effectively. This can become one of many arenas of people's power. In this broader context, the 'Right to Health-Care' and certain other health-related rights are potentially at least partially achievable in the current social framework.

However, achievement of the 'Right to Health' for all, in its fullest comprehensive sense constitutes our larger vision, which is inextricably linked with larger social transformations. Keeping this in mind, the struggle for health rights must move on to link with several other struggles for the rights to food, water, education, housing, livelihood and social justice in various forms, not only because these rights are extremely germane to the improvement of health, but also because the struggle for health rights must form one strand of a much larger struggle to challenge the dominant social order.

Establishing people's right to health-care may be one of the platforms for developing people's awareness and strength, and for beginning to shape certain incipient models of the future within the present. But a broader movement needs to take shape to present coherent alternatives in myriad spheres of life to nurture the tender saplings of the future even in the harsh world of today. Only such a movement can also dream of replacing the current unhealthy and inequitable socio-economic system, by one that is far more just, humane and healthy, in the world of tomorrow.

A Paradigm Shift: Policy Objectives for Larger Goals

With this perspective, it may be suggested to achieve policy goal for health as a right. We need to work in a co-ordinated manner towards the establishment of a system for universal access to appropriate quality health-care. A complex and difficult process of social mobilisation, policy debate and shaping of political will would be required to make such a situation part of the reality. As mentioned above, it would not be just a narrow 'demanding of existing entitlements' but would also require a broader interpretation of health rights, with a progressive redefining of entitlements.

It may be suggested that we would need to work for some of the following objectives (a demonstrative, not exhaustive list) to move towards achieving this larger goal:

- First and foremost, a considerably strengthened, accountable and reoriented public health system. Such a rejuvenation of the public health system would require changes at levels of policy, structure, programmes, and processes. Such strengthening should ensure adequate infrastructure, human power, services and supplies at various levels, restoring the basic functionality of the system and rebuilding public confidence. Mechanisms for public accountability would need to be put in place, along with reorientation of staff at various levels to rebuild their motivation and responsiveness.
- The base of strengthened public health would need to be a framework of comprehensive primary health-care including community health workers in every habitation, functional and accountable primary health centres and first referral units, combined with a range of appropriate preventive and promotive activities. The indispensability of community health workers has been noted again

and again, yet the need for strong community anchoring, flexibility and local evolution of diverse models, emphasis on empowering women, role of community representation and demand generation by CHW, and hence a strong, equitable (not top-down) linkage with the public health system needs to be considered while developing these programmes. This would need to be accompanied by a significant degree of genuine decentralization of planning (which presupposes decentralization of finances and power, not just responsibility).

- Linked with such strengthening of the public health system, to institutionalize accountability would require a legal and constitutional framework to assure health services as a right. The definition of essential services' i.e. the range of services that would be ensured for all citizens as a legal entitlement, has been an issue of severe political contentions in all countries wherever the 'universal access package' has been defined.
- The above processes would obviously necessitate mechanisms for substantially raising public finances for the public health system, through general taxation along with various forms of special taxation would cease health security. Corporations and employers in both organized and unorganized sectors would be required to contribute substantially to the general health system, even as their employees including unorganized workers receive good quality health-care coverage from a strengthened health system.
- Specific health-care requirements of various groups with special needs – such as women, children, and elderly persons – would need to be met through sets of special measures, sensitively delivered by the general health system. Women's health will have to be conceptualized and addressed in a framework

larger than reproductive health, reaching women in all stages of the life cycle, while services for the entire range of women's health issues are integrated with an upgraded general health system. All coercive measures for population control should be regarded as serious human rights violations and should be terminated. In the context of children's health and nutrition, ICDS will require universalisation, enhanced funds and staffing support, systematic linkage with the health-care and education systems, and a much greater role to the community.

- Specific major health problem, both communicable diseases such as TB and HIV-AIDS, and non-communicable health issues such as mental health would need to be addressed through programmes closely integrated with a robust comprehensive health system. These programmes integrated with the comprehensive system could subsume and replace the current selective, vertical programmes. Concerning communicable disease control, the emphasis would need to be on social-ecological methods appropriate to various diseases and situations, with involvement of communities in planning and implementation, which are presently major gaps.
- Legislation should be enacted which would control private medical sector to meet minimum standards, follow standard treatment guidelines, and observe ceilings on prices of essential health services. They may be progressively brought under the umbrella of a universal access system and may be contracted by this publicly regulated system to provide services, while the recipient of care is not required to pay while receiving these services.
- Much more effective public health support to indigenous healing systems is required, including

active research on areas such as community-based evaluation of indigenous healing methods and synergistic combination with modern medicine. The emphasis would need to be on integration of systems and creation of 'basic doctors' who can provide a range of appropriate care especially at the primary level.

- Operationalising accountability and redressal mechanisms to ensure regular civil society monitoring and inputs at various levels (village/ block/district/state/national), which would be the concrete form of the public re-entering and reclaiming the public health system. Panchayati Raj community-based organizations including women's groups could play a key role in ensuring accountability of the health system. At the same time, an effective redressal system would be required to deal with complaints and denial of health-care in various forms through responsive, and time-bound mechanisms.

In order to fulfil the mandate of health-care sector, the Ministry of Health and Family Welfare, being the central core ministry for implementing health-care activities, has taken several initiatives, some of which may be seen as follows:

It is pertinent to mention here that under the National Common Minimum Programme (NCMP) of Union Government; health-care is one of the seven thrust areas. The NCMP mandates an increase in expenditure in health sector, with main focus on Primary Health-care from the current level of 0.9% of GDP to 2-3% of GDP over the next five years. The National Rural Health Mission (NRHM) which is the main vehicle for giving effect to the above mandate was launched on 12.4.05 by Hon'ble Prime Minister of India. It has been operationalized throughout the country, with special focus on 18 states which includes eight Empowered Action Group States (Bihar, Jharkhand, Madhya Pradesh, Chhattisgarh, Uttar Pradesh, Uttarakhand, Orissa and Rajasthan), and eight North-East States, as well as Himachal Pradesh and Jammu and Kashmir.

The main aim of NRHM is to provide accessible, affordable, accountable, effective and reliable primary health-care facilities, especially, to the poor and vulnerable sections of the population. It also aims at bridging the gap in rural health-care services through creation of a cadre of Accredited Social Health Activists (ASHA) and improved hospital care, decentralization of programme to district level to improve intra- and inter-sectoral convergence and effective utilization of resources.

The NRHM further aims to provide overarching umbrella to the existing programmes of Health and Family Welfare including RCH-II, malaria, blindness, iodine deficiency, filaria, Kala-Azar, T.B., leprosy and integrated disease surveillance. Further, it addresses the issue of health in the context of sector-wide approach addressing sanitation and hygiene, nutrition and safe drinking water as basic determinants of good health in order to have greater convergence among the related social sector departments, i.e. AYUSH, Women and Child Development, Sanitation, Elementary Education, Panchayati Raj and Rural Development.

The mission further seeks to build greater ownership of the programme among the community through involvement of Panchayati Raj Institutions, NGOs and other stake holders at national, state, district and sub-district levels to achieve the goals of National Population Policy 2000 and National Health Policy.

Recently Govt of India has also started National Health Mission, comprising of urban and rural health care of entire country.

The vision of the mission may be seen as follows

- To provide effective healthcare to rural population throughout the country with special focus on 18 states, which have weak public health indicators and/or weak infrastructure.
- To raise public spending on health from 0.9% GDP to 2-3% of GDP, with improved arrangement for community financing and risk pooling.
- To undertake architectural correction of the health system to enable it to effectively handle increased allocations and promote policies that strengthen public health management and service delivery in the country.
- To revitalize local health traditions and mainstream AYUSH into the public health system.
- Effective integration of health concerns through decentralized management at district, with determinants of health like sanitation and hygiene, nutrition, safe drinking water, gender and social concerns.
- Address inter-state and inter district disparities.
- To emphasize the Public Private Partnerships.
- Involvement of Panchayati Raj Institutions.
- To improve access to rural people, especially poor women and children to equitable, affordable, accountable and effective primary health-care.

Flexible and decentralized planning is the pivot on which the entire concept of the mission revolves. The following points highlight the process:

- The planning process under the guidance of the Village Health and Sanitation Committee to start right from the village level. The district plans would thereafter converge into state plans.
- Planning would be taken up for the entire mission period as well as for each financial year.

- For the purpose of preparation of annual plan, in the month of October, the states would be given an indication of the quantum of funds, untied as well as those under Reproductive and Child Health – II and various vertical disease control programmes like TB, vector-borne diseases, leprosy, malaria, disease surveillance, etc. The states would in turn indicate to the districts their respective shares.
- Based on the normative framework currently being developed, the District Health Mission under the guidance of the Zilla Parishad would get the plan prepared.
- A small part of the funds at the district as well as at the state level to be set apart for taking up innovative schemes.
- Even though funds for programmes involving other determinants of health would continue to flow through their respective channel, the district health plan would incorporate the activities being taken up at the local level.
- The district plans would be appraised by the states, who thereafter would send the state plans to the Centre. These plans would be approved at the central level before the beginning of the financial year.

National vector-borne disease control programme (NVBDCP): NVBDCP is concerned with prevention and control of vector borne diseases, namely malaria, Kala-Azar, filariasis, dengu and Japanese encephalitis. The vector-born-disease are complex; since their presence and transmission depends upon interaction of numerous ecological, biological, social and economic factors. Increasing travel within and across countries is also responsible for spread of vector-borne diseases. Under NVBDCP three pronged approach for prevention and control of disease is case detection and treatment, vector management by reduction of transmission of risk and supportive intervention including behaviour change communication.

Status of Kala-Azar Elimination in Bihar

In Bihar, study on social and economic impact of Kala-Azar reveals that *VL* affects the rural poor, causing significant morbidity and mortality. High cost of diagnosis and treatment causes substantial social and economic hardship for effected families. In endemic areas, increased infection risk is mediated through poor housing conditions and environmental sanitation, lack of personal protection measures and economically driven migration and employment that bring people into contact with infected sandflies. Poverty is associated with poor nutrition and other infectious disease, which increase the risk that a person (once infected) will progress to the clinically manifested disease. Lack of health-care access causes delay in appropriate diagnosis and treatment and eventually increases leishmaniasis morbidity and mortality.

Leishmaniasis diagnosis and treatment are expensive and families must sell assets and take loans to pay for care, leading to further impoverishment and reinforcement of the vicious cycle of disease and poverty. *Visceral leishmaniasis* has a huge social impact due to lost educational potential, reduced economic productivity and stigma. *VL* results in missed days of work for adults, especially the family breadwinner. Therefore, *VL* not only occurs in the context of poverty, but through their adverse social impact they may also promote poverty. The stigmatizing nature of *VL* often causes afflicted individuals to turn away from social contact. The interruption of public health services and migrations has produced resurgences in *VL*.

□

11

Summary of Whole Issues at a Glance

It is evident from the fact and day-to-day experiences that essential components of the right to health-care must include:

1. Appropriate infrastructure in the form of sub-centers/primary health centers/community health Centers with attendant and basic facilities;
2. Skilled human resources like medical professionals and other health-care and paramedical staff rendering required range of services;
3. Medicines and supplies which are basic and essential;
4. Emergency medical care;
5. Patient information, redressal; and
6. Monitoring and professional accountability.

After careful consideration, it has been noticed that the following steps may be required for providing right to health-care:

- An innumerable number of studies and documentation in socio-economic context have clarified that lack of potable drinking water is the root cause for many of our health hazards. Undoubtedly, if governance takes appropriate measures to provide potable drinking water, millions of our population will be saved from related diseases and illnesses.

- Similarly, in case of health-care, delivery centers in the form of health centers, a lot needs to be done to make them accessible to cater to health needs.
- Availability of affordable and essential drugs is another related sphere, which warrants immediate attention from the state.
- Strategically, it is desirable to direct the judicial focus to health-care rather than health as such. Scope and ambit of health-care is relatively narrower than health, amenable to meaningful implementation of judicial orders. Accordingly, specific and precise dimensions or facets of health-care must be clearly spelt out. In addition, wherever it is required, efforts must be made to strengthen the already existing statutory guidelines or mandates or applicable judicial order.
- Instead of focusing exclusively on judicial intervention and remedies, it is necessary to initiate appropriate processes to the sensitivities of the political authorities as well. This requires a concerted action to bring health-care within political discourse. Collective efforts must be made to convince political leaders about the mileage that health issues can draw in the political processes.
- Attempts must be made to legislate the right to health-care with all its essential components, which ultimately paves the way for incorporation into our Constitution as a fundamental right.
- All non-government employees living in the rural area may be issued a Limited Paying Capacity Card, which will ensure free accessibility to all the essential medical services as is being provided to BPL card holders. This card could be issued by the local district administration.

- Need to have a recognized course for nursing practitioners to ensure availability of independent treatment and also specialists like nurses anesthetist and gynecologists in the rural parts of the country.
- The Medical Council of India and the Nursing Council of India to have a relook and work out a methodology to recognize course for nursing practitioner.
- Under NRHM, ASHA should be strengthened so that she remains not just a motivator but a Community Health Worker capable of providing basic health-care.
- Public-Private Partnerships (PPP) may be considered in one of the major intervention areas of health-care. There is a need for enacting a National Clinical Registration and Regulation Act to develop various standards to be observed even by the private institutions running health-care facilities.
- There is a need to have a proper drug procurement mechanism to ensure guaranteed availability of all essential drugs at the sub-centre, primary and secondary care level. Also, to create awareness regarding the availability of the essential drugs, the appropriate government may print a booklet having a list of essential drugs which would be necessarily available at PHC/CHC/district hospitals.
- Need to develop 'Emergency Medicines' as a specialty to improve the emergency medical services in the country.
- The maternal health services should also focus on adequate treatment of maternal anemia including safe institutional delivery services, health promotion and health education concerning safe motherhood.

- All states should enact a Public Health Act to enshrine the Health Rights of citizens related to public health services and public health conditions.
- Need to have a redressal mechanism to ensure right to health as such. Therefore, it is recommended the complaints received by the Rogi Kalyan Samiti/Monitoring Committees must be referred to the respective State Human Rights Commission.
- Need to review pulse polio based eradication strategy and to consider compensation for all children affected by Vaccine Associated Paralytic Polio.

□

Annexures

1. Matrix for Kala-Azar elimination:

Overview	
Information on Sandfly, its life cycle and possible breeding places	*Comments*
Sandfly – *P. argentipes* is a small, dark brown, hairy insect about 2.5 mms. from the tip of mouth parts to the last abdominal segment. It belongs to the sub-family *Phlebotominae* which comprises more than 600 species. Of about 50 species of sandflies present in India, *P. argentipes* is the only species that transmits Kala-Azar to man. *P. argentipes* has a very wide distribution range, stretching from Iran to Indonesia. But the core area of its distribution range lies in the, eastern and south eastern India, where because of availability of the alluvial soil, high humidities, relatively equable temperatures, abundance of cattle population, it is able to build up enormous population densities and transmit kala-azar.	Sandfly is 1/3rd the size of the mosquito and has high tendency to breed in warm and moist places and its prevalence in Bihar is attributed to the environmental factors.
Life cycle of Sandfly – The life cycle of sandflies resembles that of mosquitoes in the basic pattern. Comprise of four stages: eggs, larval,	Life cycle of sandfly is completed in the moist soil unlike mosquito which

the non-feeding pupal and the adult. However, sandflies including the vector *P. argentipes* breed in moist soil unlike mosquitoes which breed in water. The larvae after hatching out from the eggs, penetrate some inches below the surface of the substrate. The larval feed on decaying organic matters. The four larval stage, lead to progressive growth and last about 10 days. The larval stage is followed by the non-feeding pupal stage which lasts about 7-10 days under optimum conditions. The larvae are very small with body covered with numerous chaetae which glue substrate particles and mask them. That is the reason only older larvae and pupae can be found in soil samples after most careful searches. No eggs or younger larvae of sandflies have ever been found in nature. Eggs and larvae of *P. argentipes* can withstand immersion in water for considerable time. First stage larvae can survive immersion for five days, and larvae of the 4th stage for 14 days. These findings possibly explain the survival of larvae in the soil during the heavy monsoon rains when their breeding places may be flooded. Breeding places of *P. argentipes* are found within a radius of about 20 yards of a dwelling house, in dark, humid soil protected from sunlight. In the cattle sheds, the favorite breeding place is the floor underneath the earthenware trough. *P. argentipes* does not breed in rodent burrows, outside or in the dwellings. After emergence the adults feed and	breeds in water. Because of this, the anti-larval insecticides or other chemical and biological control methods used in mosquito control cannot be applied to sandfly. Moreover, due to high fertile land in Bihar and flooding, especially water-logging for a long period because of poor drainage system constitutes the whole land favourable for the breeding of the sandfly. Feeding on the plant juices during the pre-transmission period is again favourable by the greeneries found in Bihar.

mate within about 24-48 hours. The males often form swarms on buffaloes seeking mating females. Female sandflies require a blood meal for egg development and maintenance of water balance. They also imbibe plant juices, a fact of considerable epidemiological importance as the capacity of *Phlebotomus* argentipes to transmit *L. donovani* is enhanced by feeding plant juices. Only the female sandflies are haematophagous, i.e. take a blood meal. *Phlebotomus argentipes* prefers cattle blood to human. But during the transmission season from June to October, when there is tremendous build up of *P. argentipes* densities there is a spill over of population into human dwellings, enhancing man-vector contact. During feeding, saliva is introduced into the host, one component of which is a peptide considered to be one of the most potent vasodilators ever discovered. Sandfly saliva enhances the growth of Leishmania in the host. In the Assam state, and adjoining plains of the north-eastern India, *P. argentipes*, has apparently been eliminated by continuous anti-malaria spraying. In these states no indigenous Kala-Azar has been reported since the 1950's except in year 2005 when one case was reported from State of Assam. In addition to blood, sandflies also ingest cells lying in the dermis outside the blood circulation and thus infected macrophages may be picked up.	

Resting places Adult sandflies are active after the dusk hours. During daytime they escape into their resting shelters. These shelters are protected from sunlight, excessive temperature. In the Kala-Azar endemic areas of India, *P. argentipes* is entirely endophilic (indoor resting and feeding). Among thousand of *P. argentipes* collected, from Bihar and Jharkhand, only one male specimen was collected from an outdoor rodent burrow. This fact is very important from the point of view of Kala-Azar elimination. A vector species with little variation in resting places can be easily targeted for residual insecticidal spraying. The presence of large numbers of *P. argentipes* on the lower margins of walls of mud houses is attributable to lot of moisture on the lower side of the dwellings. High humidities are a decisive factor in the life history of *P. argentipes* is active in humidity range of 75-85%. This is the main reason why it is abundant during monsoon and post-monsoon seasons. Development of mature eggs, after taking a blood (gonotrophic cycle) is completed in about 3-4 days time. Sandflies must take at least two blood meals to transmit leishmania to man. Thus, the presence of parous sandflies (which has laid at least one batch of eggs) in a population of sandflies is important to know the potentially infective flies. Determination of the age of the sandflies is also important in assessing the effectiveness of treatment with insecticides. Ovaries of nulliparous (not laid eggs) females resemble a compact bunch of grapes. The follicles (precursors of eggs) are	Sandfly is nocturnal and endophilic and makes it an easy target for sprays. One male species is outdoor, but information regarding its transmissibility has to be obtained. Since females are hemophilus, there is a high possibility of outdoor species to be non-transmissible for Kala-Azar. However, nothing can be stated at this point of time. Indoor Residual Spray remains the only chemical method to control sandfly.

very compact and do not move far from each other when pressed under a cover slip. The ovaries of parous females when pressed under a microscope cannot contract for a long time and remain in an extended form. They appear loose and covered with a light net. A small number of mature eggs with undeveloped follicles and an empty stomach indicates that this female had laid at least one batch of eggs. The accessory glands of the oviducts produce a secretion containing numerous granules. In the newly hatched female, the glands are nearly empty with no granules. The granules appear only after the first blood meal. Females with no or few granules in the glands are newly hatched individuals, while females without a trace of blood in the stomach, with eggs in the early stage of development, but with granules in the accessory glands, are individuals which have digested a blood meals and laid a batch of eggs.	
Dispersal of sandflies The dispersal range of *P. argentipes* is restricted to about 25 metres. It is a poor flier, moving in short hopping flights. **Seasonal Dynamics** High densities of *P. argentipes* are a pre-requisite for Kala-Azar transmission. Transmission season of Kala-Azar in India is coincident with the season of the highest *P. argentipes* densities, and which is from June to October. In the north-east India, *P. argentipes* vanishes in the cold months of December and January and reappears in small numbers in March. The numbers shoot up dramatically after the onset of monsoon and remain high till the end of October	Sandfly can move upto 25 metres and lives within 60 feet of the human dwellings. It disappears in December and January. The areas for IRS should take these two factors in consideration.

Matrix for Life Cycle Stages of Sandfly According to the Outputs

Life Cycle Stages	*Output 1*	*Output 2*	*Output 3*	*Output 4*	*Output 5*	*Timings*	
Increase scale and functionality	Community participation	System strengthening	NGOs	Monitoring and evaluation		March	
Eggs		making the soil dry by putting some dry matter or cementing the surroundings (moist soil)				March-April	Little information is known about these and the only
Jarva		removing all organic debris and making the soil dry and cementing the surrounding (feed on organic matter)			measures available may be extremely difficult.	March-April	
Pupa		making the soil dry (found in wet soil)				March-April	

Adult		Filling all cracks and crevices within 20 yards of any human dwellings, mobilising all the cattle, disposal of cow dung as soon as it excretes and dry it in the roof before the evening, removing all plants within 20 yards of human dwellings, drying the soil beneath in the cattle shed, keeping buffaloes away at the distance of 25 metres of human dwellings, DDT Spraying on plants, keeping the cows in ITBNs at night				March-June	Targeting the breeding the restling places of sandfly are the only measures taken at this place.

BCC for passive case detection, BCC for effectiveness of IRS		involving NGOs for BCC			March-June	
ITBN for each Kala-Azar patient at each facility		the person sleeping in cattle-shed is slept at the height of 6 feet, each person using ITBN (to avoid sandfly bite), manual collection of sandfly by trained personnels, killing by light traps, collection and killing by sticky paper traps, regular cleaning of houses and sheds before night, filling up the cracks and crevices, fuming at late evening and night Training of spray workers, Training of Mos and ANMs for spray monitoring			June-October	These measures shall be helpful in preventing sandfly-human contact to limited extent and some (ITBN) might even decrease the sandfly to some extent. However, these alone (without IRS) are not sufficient to control sandfly.

2. Road map for Kala-Azar Elimination:

Overview of Kala-Azar Situation in Bihar

Kala-Azar – Kala-Azar is endemic in 33 out of 38 districts in Bihar. Non-endemic districts are Kaimur, Rohtas, Gaya, Aurangabad and Jamui. As of year 2011 with data upto November 2011, 23848 cases out of 31322 cases in India, are found in Bihar with 74 deaths out of 78 in India. Kala-Azar Control Programme was started in 1992. It is centrally funded and now is being financially supported by World Bank. There are multiple challenges affecting the Kala-Azar Elimination Program.

1. Under reporting of cases and deaths
2. Lack of awareness in the community
3. Unmotivated Health Department
4. Low incentives to ASHAs
5. No Quality Monitoring of IRS
6. DDT resistance in some districts
7. Lack of knowledge on all the possible breeding sites and life cycle of sandfly
8. Poverty and Malnutrition
9. Prolonged treatment
10. Asymptomatic cases
11. PKDL cases (asymptomatic carriers)
12. HIV and TB coinfected cases
13. No proper referral system
14. No proper Active Case Search

Overview of Kala-Azar Elimination Roadmap for DFID-SWASTH: DFID SWASTH is providing technical assistance to Government of Bihar in eliminating Kala-Azar along with TB and Maternal and Child Health Services Improvement. The following roadmap has been prepared by disease Control Wing of SWASTH. The roadmap aims to achieve elimination goal by 2020 and prioritizes prevention of deaths and then subsequent elimination efforts.

1. Prevention of Deaths: Death prevention is based on the studies on Kala-Azar cases, according to which,

Prognosis of Kala-Azar Treated cases in India is almost 100%. Thus, efforts are centered to strengthen passive surveillance through community and ASHA sensitization and active surveillance by actively searching each patient of Kala-Azar and ensuring that the patient is completely treated (cured). Since ASHAs are the platforms between health and community and the roadmap starts with the sensitization of ASHAs for proper case detection. In addition, capacity building of MOs and ANMs are essential in order to improve the treatment and programme management part of Medical staff. The other activities involve sensitization of community by these health professionals and filling the gaps in the treatment part. The roadmap also aims at strengthening of some specialized centers for special cases of Kala-Azar not managed at three levels of healthcare and their referral to these centers.

2. Elimination of Kala-Azar: Elimination strategies incorporates, in addition to the above activities, hygiene and other physical methods to prevent sandfly-human contact. There is a provision of strict quality monitoring and assurance of Indoor Residual Spray. Data mapping has to be done (strategies for that are mentioned in next tab). Since community involvement is vital to Kala-Azar eradication, a "Community Voucher Scheme" has been designed to actively involve community in Kala-Azar Control. A study undertaken by PHFI and supported by DFID has been chosen which will measure DDT resistance and quality control of IRS and shall be able to provide expert recommendations on elimination of Kala-Azar. In addition, a study has been proposed to bring more light to life cycle of sandfly and possible interventional measures that will be useful to eradicate sandfly.

3. Final Elimination strategies: The final strategy will include an elimination team which will actively search for sandfly and symptomatic and asymptomatic cases for any isolated case. The team will target the residual resting and breeding places of sandfly using different methods.

Roadmap for Kala-Azar Elimination by Year 2020

Goals	*Measures*	*Activities*	*Year*	*Outputs (timelines)*	*Things*	*Needed*	*Roles*	*Outcome expected*
Prevent deaths	(Based on the finding that the survival rate of patients treated is nearly 98% – Goal is to ensure that each patient is diagnosed early and treated completely and complicated cases are dealt in a special way) Strengthening							
	Surveillance	1. Capacity Building of ASHAs (two times in a year before each IRS) 2. Capacity Building of Mos in phased manner (highly endemic and then endemic) 3. Capacity Building of ANMs through IEC (33 endemic districts)	2014-16	Output 3			D. Partners/NGOs state and district teams	Reporting increased, Health Staff Motivated for Kala-Azar elimination and treatment. medical officers motivated to take active participation in Kala-Azar control programme (Efforts for strengthening Active surveillance)
	Increasing Community awareness for case detection	1. Sensitization through ASHAs 2. Sensitization through MOs 3. Sensitization through VBD staff	2014-15 2014-15 2014-15	Output 2			D. Partners/NGOs state and district teams	Reporting increased, Community sensitized and efforts made that each case is

		4. Community Voucher Scheme 5. BCC strategy in community voucher scheme 6. Scaling it up in the whole state in phases 7. Hoardings in selected sites	2014-2016 2014-16				reported and treated completely. (efforts to increase passive surveillance)
	Ensuring Availability of Diagnostic and treatment facilities at each facility and their strengthening KTS	For all cases and 1. DOTS for Miltefosine 2. Referral arrangement 3. Follow-up of cases for treatment compliance by	2014-16	Output 1	1. DOTS trial for drug compliance 2. Incentive for referral 3. Special Diet or Some Iron to supplementation for Kala-Azar patients	D. Partners/NGOs state and district teams	Improving diagnostic and treatment facilities, ensuring complete drug compliance, preventing deaths or complications due to anemia.
	Strengthening of specialized facilities for diagnostic and treatment facilities	For PKDL, HIV/TB, malnourished and complicated cases	2014-16	Output 1	Transmission pattern and rates	Govt, World Bank and MSF	Identifying and managing special cases

For Elimination	Strengthening Surveillance	1. Active Case Search Strengthening 2. Mapping of the cluster of cases 3. Strategies in different areas based on cases and DDT resistance and recommendations for getting it done at right time and right way	2014-15	Output 3	Mapping of cases at state, district, block and village levels	D. Partners/NGOs state and district teams	Identifying areas of high priorities and strategies adopted in these areas.
	Hygiene and Other Measures (filling up cracks and crevices, ITBN, etc.) – part of community voucher scheme	1. Pilot in one district 2. Scaling it up to the whole state in phased manner	2014-15 2014-16	output 2		D. Partners/NGOs state and district teams	Additional measures to prevent human-sandfly contact for its control and their effects assessed.
	IRS	1. Pilot for monitoring of IRS quality in one area by community (Kushal Club, SHGs,	2014-15	Output 2		D. Partners/NGOs state and district teams	Quality improvement in IRS

		youth clubs, etc.) in community voucher scheme					
		2. Scaling it up in the whole state in phased manner	2014-16	output 3		D. Partners/N GOs state and	
		3. Study for resistance against DDT and recommendations for use of another insecticide in the sprays and quality assurance of IRS (Institutional Study)	2014-15	Output 5		D. Partners/N GOs state and district teams	Extent of DDT resistance assessed and technical aspects of quality assurance of IRS revised.
		4. Findings of Institutional study to be shared with the govt. and recommendations provided to govt.	2014-15	Output 5		D. Partners/N GOs state and district teams	
	Additional Studies finding an	1. Study on Life Cycle of Sandfly and intervention 2. Piloting in one district	2014-16	Output 5 sandfly and	Information on life cycle of some interventions	D. Partners/N GOs state and district teams	More information on life cycle of sandfly gathered and an intervention added to

		3. Scaling it up in the whole state					eradicate sandfly
		The above Activities should continue till 2018					
	Final Elimination Measures	Formation of an elimination team plan	2018		Team members, mapping of sites and their time	Govt.	
	Tracking Residual Cases	Active Case Detection on a mass scale	2018 – 20		Mapping of inaccessible areas and community	Govt.	Efforts to find out residual cases (symptomatic and asymptomatic cases)
	Handling residual sandfly	Fogging on a mass scale (1 species is outdoor) or aggressive IRS in houses and cattlesheds	2018-20		Does that species transmit Kala-Azar	Govt.	To be decided to damage all possible breeding sites of sandfly
	Damaging residual breeding places	Identification and eradication of pockets of sandfly breeding places by multiple methods by a specialized team	2018-20		All possible breeding places of sandfly	Govt.	Residual sandflies destroyed

3. Strategies for Kala-Azar Elimination:

<table>
<tr><td colspan="2">Overview of Strategies – A data mapping needs to be done in all areas of prevalence of Kala-Azar based on the number of cases and DDT resistance. The data needs to be divided into three areas and different interventions need to be employed in each of these.</td></tr>
<tr><th colspan="2">Strategies to be implemented according to the endemicity</th></tr>
<tr><td>Area 1 (high cases and high DDT resistance) or high DDT resistance</td><td>1. Community sensitization by Voucher Scheme and KTS
2. IRS with alternate insecticide or mixed insecticides
3. Active Case Search (at least two times in a year on mass scale and regular in camp modes)
4. Annual data mapping based on the search
5. Hoardings at public places
6. BCC strategy for IRS and Active case search
7. IEC for each Facility
8. Sensitization of ASHAs for Active case search</td></tr>
<tr><td>Area 2 (high cases and little or no resistance)</td><td>1. Community voucher scheme
2. Active Case Search in regular camp modes
3. Active community sensitization by all means
4. Annual data mapping of cases
5. BCC strategy for active case search</td></tr>
<tr><td>Area 3 (low cases or no cases)</td><td>1. Surveillance and strengthening of diagnostic and treatment facilities
2. Hygiene and other practices</td></tr>
</table>

4. Environmental and Social Hindrances in Kala-Azar Elimination:

Overview of major environmental and social factors affecting Kala-Azar elimination – There are some Environmental and social factors hindering the effective implementation of Kala-Azar elimination. These challenges need to be taken care of, and issues needs to be addressed by government combined with the Kala-Azar elimination initiatives for successful implementation of program.	
Major Challenges in eradicating sandfly or elimination of Kala-azar	*Comments*
1. **Flood and water logging during the period of transmission**	Flooding is common in Bihar and occurs especially in the Monsoon and post-monsoon season, which co-incides with the peak season of transmission of Kala-Azar. Moreover, large amount of land remains water-logged for a considerably longer period of time. Sandfly gets the best environment for its breeding and multiplication. Since lots of areas are submerged, Indoor Residual Spray does not take place at places which is most favorable for sandfly breeding. There is a recommendation to improve drainage system and to spray these areas with some special team.
2. **Environment extremely suitable (fertile land and humidity 75-85%) for sandfly breeding**	Extremely suitable natural environment makes it difficult to eradicate sandfly, and according to

	Theory of Natural Selection, there is a possibility of sandfly changing its breeding places. Hence, there is a recommendation of fogging in combination with IRS during its last elimination phase in case that happens.
3. **Customary habits of indigenous people (sleeping of cattle-sheds) and cow-dung regarded as the holy thing.**	Old customs are very difficult to change. People in Bihar sleep in cattle-shed to protect their cattles and are primarily exposed to sandfly. Cow-dung is considered as a holy thing by the indigenous people which is a preferential breeding site of sandfly in Bihar. Educating the people regarding the ill-effects of dung will have to be dealt with very cautiously and intelligently. Still, BCC for this will remain a challenge.
4. ***Kachcha* Houses and plenty of breeding sites of sandfly in such houses.**	Kachcha house in rainy season without the flood, is itself a favourable breeding site with multiple crevices and cracks and in floods the situation becomes grave. There should be a provision to launch some housing schemes in areas of high prevalence of Kala-Azar

	and *pucca* houses should be provided to the people in such areas.
5. Very little known about the life cycle of sandfly guidelines for vector.	No eggs or early larvae have ever been discovered in nature (taken from control at www.nvbdcp.org). There is an information required to find out more about the life cycle and possible interventions to be included in Kala-Azar elimination.
6. No information of all the breeding places of sandfly.	There should be an aggressive search for all the possible breeding sites of sandfly.
7. Poverty and Malnutrition in Bihar	Kala-Azar is a disease mainly affecting the poor people and becomes deadly because many of them are malnourished too. There is a need to.
8. Poor sanitation and education	Poor sanitary habits and illiteracy needs to be improved. Progressive efforts should be built up towards that by GoB.
9. Indoor Residual Spray Guidelines	Current guidelines for targeting villages under IRS are 1 case/village for the last five years. However, the sandfly moves with the migrating population and many a times the neighbouring villages suspected of having sandfly are not

	sprayed. This focal spraying leads to hidden built-up of sandfly in neighbouring villages. There is a need to revise the guidelines and all for a possible areas surrounding any village affected of Kala-Azar should be sprayed or as raised several times in many national level meetings, the whole state of Bihar should be sprayed simultaneously.

□

References

www.nvbdcp.org – signs and symptoms of Kala-Azar.

Addy, M., Mitro, A.K., Ghosh, K.K., Hati, A.K. (1983). Host preference of *P. argentipes* in different biotopes. *Trop. Geogr Med. 35:* 343-45.

Adler, S. and Theodor, O. (1957). Transmission of disease agents by Phlebotomine sandflies. *Ann. Rev. Ento. 2:* 203-206.

Alder and P. Theodor. [Study of bionomics of Phlebotomine sandflies.] *J. Insect Sci. (1986).*

Alvar, J., Canavate, C., Gutierrez-Solar, B., Jimenez, M., Laguna, F., Lopez-Velez, R., *et al.* Leishmania and human immunodeficiency virus coinfection: the first 10 years. *Clin Microbiol Rev,* 1997; 10: 298-319.

Alvar, J., Yactayo. S., Bern, C. Leishmaniasis and poverty. *Trends Parasitol,* 2006; *22*(12): 552-57.

Amalraj, D.D., Sivagnaname, N. and Srinivasan, R. (1999). Susceptibility of *Phlebotomus argentipes* and *P. papatasi* (Diptera: Psychodidae) to insecticides. *J. Commun. Dis. 31:* 177-180.

Ansari, M.A. and Rajdan, R.K. Operational feasibility of malaria control by burning neem oil in kerosene lamp in Beel Akbarpur village, district Ghaziabad. *Indian J Malariol., 33:* 81.

Ansari, M.A., Vasudevan, P., Tandon, M. and Razdan, R.K. Larvicidal and mosquito repellent action of peppermint (*Mentha piperita*) oil. *Bioresource Technol 71:* 267, 1999.

Azeez, S.A. (1964). Susceptibility Status of *An. Fluiatilis* and *An. Annularis* to DDT in an area near Dhanbad. *Bull.Soc. Mal. Dis., 1:* 53-54.

Basak, B. and N. Tandon (1995). Observations on susceptibility status of *Phlebotomus argentipes* to DDT in District South 24-Paraganas, West Bengal. *J.Commun. Dis.,* 196-197.

Batra, C.P., Mittal, P.K., Adak, T. and Sharma, V.P. Efficacy of neem-water emulsion against mosquito immatures. *Indian J Malariol, 35:* 15, 1998.

Bern, C., Chowdhury, R. The epidemiology of visceral leishmaniasis in Bangladesh: Prospects for improved control. *Indian J Med Res,* 2006; *123:* 275-88.

Bern, C., Jha, S.N., Joshi, A.B., Thakur, G.D., Bista, M.B. Use of the recombinant k39 dipstick test and the direct agglutination test in a setting endemic for visceral leishmaniasis in Nepal. *Am J Trop Med Hyg,* 2000; 63: 153-57.

Brahmchari, U.N. Treatise on Kala-Azar *(John Bale and Dannielson Ltd., London),* 1928.

Buttiker, W., An improved sampling method for phlebotomine sandflies developed in Saudi Arabia. *Mitt Schweiz Ent Ges, 52:* (1979) 117.

Campbell, F.L., Sullivan, W.W. and Smith, L.N. (1993). The relative toxicity of nicotine, anabasine, methyl anabasine and lupipine for culicine mosquito larvae. *J Econ Entomol, 26:* 500, 1993.

Cerf, B.J., Jones, T.C., Badaro, R., Sampaio, D., Teixeira, R., Johnson, W.D. Jr. Malnutrition as a risk factor for severe visceral leishmaniasis. *J Infect Dis* 1987; 156: 1030-33.

Chaika, S.Y. (1975). Electron microscopic investigation of the olfactory sensilla of the sandfly *Phlebotomus papatasi* (Diptera: Phlebotomidae); in Proceedings of the 2nd all-Union symposium on insect chemoreception, *Vilnus,* pp 6975.

Chandra, Gautam, Bhattacharya, J. and Hati, A.K. (1995). Susceptibility status of *Phlebotomus argentipes* to DDT, dieldrin and malathion in Hoogly, West Bengal. *J. Commun. Dis., 27(4):* 247-49.

Chaniotis, B.N. (1967). The biology of California *Phlebotomus* (Diptrea: Psychodidae) under laboratory conditions. *J. Med. Ent., 4,* 221-233.

Christophers, S.R., Short, H.E. and Barraud, P.J., (1926). The anatomy of the sandfly *Phlebotomus* argentipes Annadale and Brunetti (Diptera). *Indian Med. Res. Mem. 4:* 177-204.

Communicable diseases: Kala-Azar status in SEA region 2005 (online). Available at URL http://www.searo.who.int/en/Section10/Section2163.htm

Davis N.T. (1967). Leishmaniasis in the Sudan Republic. 28. Anatomical studies on *Phlebotomus orientalis* Parrot and *P. papatasi* Scopoli (Diptera: Psychodidae). *J M Entomol, 4:* 50-65.

Dellinger, D.L. (1986). Dormansy in tropical insects. *Ann. Rev. Ento., 31,* 239-64.

Deobhankar, R.B. and N.D. Palkar. Magnitude of DDT resistance in anopheles culicifarcies in Maharashtra state. *J. Commun. Dis. 32:* 65-66.

Dergacheva, T.I., Zherikhina, I.I. and Rasnitsyna, N.M. A method of counting sandflies (Diptera, Phlebotomidae). *WHO/LEISH/79,* 1979, p. 3.

Desjeux, P. Global control and Leishmania HIV co-infection. *Clin Dermatol* 1999; *17*: 317-25.

Desjeux, P. Human leishmaniases: Epidemiology and public health aspects. *World Health Stat Q,* 1992; *45*(2-3): 267-75.

Desjeux, P. Leishmaniasis: Public health aspects and control. *Clin Dermatol,* 1996; *14:* 417-23.

Desjeux, P. The increase in risk factors for leishmaniasis worldwide. *Trans R Soc Trop Med Hyg,* 2001; *95:* 239-43.

Dhanda, V., Shetty, P.S. and Dhiman, R.C. (1983). Studies on Phlebotomine sandflies as vectors of Kala-Azar in Bihar. *Proc. of Indo-UK Workshop on Leishmaniasis,* ICMR, New Delhi.

Dua, V.K., Nagpal, B.N. and Sharma, V.P. (1995). Repellent action of neem cream against mosquitoes. *Indian J. Malariol. 32: 47, 1995.*

El Saffi, S.H. and Evans, D.A. (1989). A comparison of the direct agglutination test and enzyme linked immunoabsorbant assay in the serodiagnosis of leishmaniasis in Sudan. Tra. Royal Society of Tropical Medicine and Hygiene. *83:* 334-37.

Fairchild, G.B. (1955). The relationship and classification of the Phlebotomine; *Ann. Entomol. Soc. Am., 48:* 182-196.

Frankenburg, S., Londner, M.V., Schlein, Y. and Schnur, L.F. (1985). The development of a solid phase radioimmunoassay for the detection of leishmanial parasites in the sandfly. *Amer. Jour. of Tropical Medicine and Hygiene, 34:* 266-269.

Gebre-Michael, T., Lane, R.P., Frame, I.A. and Miles, M.A. (1993). *Leishmania donovani* infection in phlebotomine sandflies from the Kala-Azar focus at Aba Roba in Ethiopia: DNA probe compared with conventional detection methods. *Medical and Veterinary Entomology*, 7 294-96.

George, J.E., (1970). Isolation of *Phlebotomus* fever from *Phlebotomus papatasi* and determination of host ranges of sandflies (Diptera: Psychodidae) in W. Pakistan. *J. Med. Ent. 7,* 670-676.

Gladwell, Malcolm (July 2, 2001). "The Mosquito Killer". The New Yorker.] [South Africa's War against Malaria Lessons for the Developing World, Richard Tren and Roger Bate, Cato Institute].

Govt. of India (2006), Annual Report 2005-06, Ministry of Health and Family Welfare, New Delhi.

Hallberg, E., Hansson, B.S. and Steinbrecht, R.A. (1944). Morphological characteristics of antennal sensilla in the Europian cornborer Ostrinia nubilalis. *Tissue Cell, 26:* 489-502.

Hati, A.K., Tandon, Neelam, Sur, S. and De, N. (1987). Exit and entrance activities of *Phlebotomus argentipes* Anandale and Brunetti, in human habitations and cowsheds. *Indian Journal of Medical Research, 86: 610-13.*

Hati, AK., Palit, A., Chakraborty, S., Bhattacharya, S., Ghosh, KK., Das, S. (1984). *Phlebotomus* argentipes caught on man baits at night in a clean isotope. *Rec. Zool. Serv. India. 81: 9-12.*

Ho, M., Siongok, T.K., Lyerly, W.H., Smith, D.H. Prevalence and disease spectrum in a new focus of visceral leishmaniasis in Kenya. *Trans R Soc Trop Med Hyg* 1982; *76:* 741-46.

http://worldhealthpartners.org/

http://www.biharvha.org/

Hurlbert SH. (1971). The non-concept of species diversity : A critique and alternative parameters: *Ecology 52: 577.*

ICMR Bulletin (2003). Prospects of using herbal products in the control of mosquito vectors. Vol. Vol. 33, No. 1 pp. 1-12.

Ilango, K., Dhanda, V., Sriniwasan, R., Sadanand, A.V. and Lane, R.P. (1944). Phlebotomine sandflies (Diptera: Psychodidae) of Tamil Nadu and Pondicherry, southern India, in relation to leishmaniasis; *Ann. Trop. Med. Parasitol., 88:* 413-431.

In Malaria War, South Africa Turns To Pesticide Long Banned in the West, Roger Thurow, *Wall Street Journal*, July 26, 2001]. [DDT and Africa's war on malaria, BBC], [Mabaso, M.L., Sharp, B., Lengeler, C. (2004). "Historical review of malarial control in southern African with emphasis on the use of indoor residual house-spraying". *Trop. Med. Int. Health 9* (8): 846-56. doi:10.1111/j.1365-3156.2004.01263.x. PMID 15303988.] [Control of Malaria Vectors in Africa and Asia C.F.Curtis].

Jha T.K., Sundar, S., Thakur, C.P., Bachmann, P., Karbwang, J., Fischer, C., *et al.* Miltefosine, an oral agent, for the treatment of Indian visceral leishmaniasis. *N Engl J Med* 1999; *341:* 1795-800.

Jobling, B. (1987). Anatomical drawings of biting flies. (London: British Museum, Natural History and the Wellcome Trust).

K. Kishore, V. Kumar, S. Keshari, D.S. Dinesh, A. Palit, C.S. Lal, A. Ranjan and S.K. Bhattacharya. (2001). Malathion slow released emulsified suspension as an effective weapon against Phlebotomine flies – A pilot study. Proceedings of *WHO Workshop* Dec. 27-28, 2001 Balaji U. Sansthan,(RMRI) Patna. p. 117-121.

Kala-Azar Commission report (Supplementary), p. 3.

Kala-Azar Commission Reports 1and 2, *Indian Medical Research Memoirs, No. 4 and No. 26* (1926, 1932).

Kalra, N.L. and Bang, Y.H. (1988). Manual on entomology in *Visceral Leishmaniasis. WHO. South-east Asia region.* p. 24.

Kalra, N.L., Kaushal Kumar and Rehman, S.J. (1986). Sandflies of Bird Tunnels in Earthen Mounds from Distt. Rohtak, (Haryana). *J. Commun. Dis., 18:* 136-138.

Kar, S.K., Ranjan, A. and Palit, A. (1999). Epidemiology of Kala-Azar in India. In: *Kala-Azar*. New Delhi: Ranbaxy

Science Foundation, Round Table Conference series, no. 5 pp. 1526.

Kaul, S.M., Chakravarty, A.K., Wattal, B.L. (1979). Record of flagellate infection in Sergentomiya sandflies in some Kala-Azar endemic areas of Bihar. *J.Com.Dis. 11, 224-225.*

Kaul, S.M., Das, R.K., Shivraj, N.B.L. Saxena and M.V.*V.L.* Narsimham (1993). Entomologicalmonitoring of Kala-Azar control in Bihar, India. Observations in Vaishali and Patna district. *J. Commun. Dis. 25(3):* 101-106.

Kaushal Kumar (1982). NICD, New Delhi/India. Annual Report.

Kaushal Kumar, Rehman, S.J., Singh, K. and Rajagopal, R. (1986). Biology of *Phlebotomus* and Sergentomia group of sandflies under laboratory conditions. *J. Com. Dis. 18:* 45-50.

Keshari, S., Palit, A., and Kishore, K. (1992). Study of breeding habitats of sandflies- Preliminary approach. *Journal of Communicable Diseases, 24 (1):* 62-63.

Killick-Kendrick, R., Investigation of phlebotomine sandflies vectors of leishmaniasis. *Proceedings of the Indo-UK Workshop on Leishmaniasis,* p. 72-83.

Killick-Kendrick, R., Leaney, A.J. and Ready, P.D. The establishment, maintenance and productivity of a laboratory colony of Lutzomyia longipalpis (Diptera: Psychodidae). *J. Med. Entomol., 13:* (1983) 429.

Krebs, C.J. (1989). Ecological methodology. (*Melano Park, CA: Addition Wesley Longman).*

Kumar, V., Keshari, S.K., Sinha, N.K., Palit, A., Kishore, K. (1995). Field trial of an ecological approach for the control of *Phlebotomus argentipes* using mud and lime laster. *Indian J. Med. Res. (A) 101:* 154-156.

Lainson R. (1983). The leishmaniasis as a global public health problem. *Proceedings of the Indo-UK Workshop on Leishmaniasis,* p. 20-35.

Lal, S.L., Bimal, S., Gupta, A.K., Sinha, S.P., Singha, U.K. and Saran, R. (1992). Serological survey of *Visceral leishmaniasis* in an epidemic village of Bihar. *Indian Journal of Comparative Microbiology, Immunology and Infectious Diseases,* 13: 28-30.

Legendre, M. Gilbert,K.J. and Witherspoon, J.G. (2005). Analyzing beta diversity : methods and implications, *Ecological Monograph, 63:* 1225.

Lewis, D.J. (1973). Phlebotomidae and Psychodidae (sandflies and moth-flies). In : Insects and other arthropods of medical importance, KGV Smith, *(Ed. Trustees of the British Museum, Natural History, London)* p. 155.

Lewis, D.J. (1975). Functional morphology of mouthparts in New world Phlebotomine sandflies. *Trans. R. Ento. Soc. Lord. B. 187: 409-19.*

Lewis, D.J. (1978). The Phlebotomine sandflies of the Oriental region. *Ento. Series. 37(6),* Bull British Museum, London.

Lewis, D.J. and Lane, R.P. (1976). A taxonomic review of *Phlebotomus* (Idio*phlebotomus*) (Psychodidae); *Syst. Entomol., 1:* 50-53.

Lowry, O.H., Rosebrough, N.J., Ferare, A. and Randdall, R.J. (1951). Protein measurement with the phenol reagent. *Journal of Biological Chemistry, 193:* 265-75.

Magurran, A.E. *Measuring biological diversity* (Oxford; Blackwell).

Margalef, R., (1958). Information theory in ecology: *Gen. Syst. 3:* 36.

Marwaha, N., Sarode, R., Gupta, R.K., Grewal, G., and Dash, S. (1991). Clinico-hematological characteristics in patients with Kala-Azar: a study from north-west India. *Trop Geogr Med 43:* 357-62.

Minter, D.M. et al. (1971). The preservation in liquid nitrogen of tsese flies and phlebotomine sandflies. *Trans. R. Soc. Trop. Med. Hyg. 65:* 175.

Mittal, P.K. and Subbarao, S.K. (2003). Prospects of using herbal products in the control of mosquito vectors. Vol. 33, No. 1 pp. 1-10.

Mittal, P.K., Adak, T. and Sharma, V.P. (1995) Bioefficacy of six neem (*Azadirachta indica*) products against mosquito larvae. *Pestic res. J. 7:* 35, 1995.

Modi, G.B. and Tesh, R.B. (1983). A simple technique for mass rearing Lutzomiya longipalpis and *Phlebotomus papatasi J. Med. Entomol., 20,* 568-569.

Molina, R. (1991). Experimental infections of a *Phlebotomus perniciosus* colony using different procedures. *Parasitologia, 33 (Suppl. 1),* 425-29.

Mubayi, A., Castillo-Chavez, C., Chowell, G., Kribs-Zaleta, C., Siddiqui, N.A., Kumar, N., Das, P. Transmission dynamics and underreporting of Kala-Azar in the Indian state of Bihar. *J Theor Biol.* 2010; *262:* 177-185.

Mukhopadhyay, A.K., Saxena, N.B.L., and Narsimham M.V.V.L. (1990). Susceptibility of *Phlebotomus argentipes* to DDT in some Kala-Azar endemic areas of Bihar (India). *Indian J. Med. Res., 91:* 458-460.

Napier LE, Dasgupta CR. An epidemiological investigation of Kala-Azar in rural areas in Bengal. Indian J Med. Res. 1931; 19: 295-341.

Napier, L.E. (1926). An epidemiological consideration of the transmission of Kala-Azar in India. *Ind. Med. Res. Memoir, 4:* 219-265.

NMEP (1990). Annual report of the National Malaria Eradication Programme, Ministry of Health and Family Welfare. India: 15-54.

Palit, A., Chawdhary, D.K. and Hati, A.K. (1988). Preliminary observation on dispersion of *P. argentipes.* (Ann. and Brun.), *I.J. parasitol., 12(1):* 15-16.

Palit, A., Kishore, K. and Sen, A.B., Gonotropic cycle of *P. argentipes* in nature in Bihar-preliminary experiences. *I. J. Parasitol. 14(2):* 121-123.

Pandya, A.P., Mehta, N.R. and Niyogi, A.K. (1975). The development of resistance in sandfly to hydrocarbon insecticides in Gujrat State. *Journal of the Indian Association of Preventive and Social Medicine,* Annual Number 111-114.

Parija, S.C. *Textbook of Medical Parasitology.* 1st ed. Chennai, India: All India Publishers and Distributors; 1996, p. 83.

Pathak et. el. (2000). Effects of few plant derived extracts on *Anopheles sp., Culex sp.* and *Ades sp. J. Medical Ento.*

Pathak, N., Mittal, P.K., Singh, O.P., Vidya Sagar and Vasudevan, P. Larvicidal action of essential oils from plants against the vector mosquitoes *Anopheles stephensi (Liston), Culex quinquefasciatus (Say) and Aedes aegypti (L). Int Pest Cont. 42:* 53, 2000.

Perich, J. and Tyagi, M. (1994). Effects of *A. indica* essential oil as repellent of some mosquitoes. *Programme on Malaria research.* 176-77.

Peters, W. and Prassad, L.S.N. (1983). Kala-Azar in India—its importance as an issue in public health. *Proceedings of the Indo-UK Workshop on Leishmaniasis,* p. 5-9.

Pillai, M.K.K. (1996). Vector resistance to insecticides. *Proc. Nat. Acad. Sci. India. 68(B)* Special Issue: 77-97.

Prince, J.D. and Rogers, L. (1914). The uniform suçcess of segregation measures in eradicating Kala-Azar for Assam tea gardens. *Brit. Med. J.I.,* 285-89.

Quate, L.W. (1964). Phlebotomine sandflies of the Paloich area in the Sudan. *J. Med. Ento., 1:* 213-68.

Ramesh, V., Mukherjee, A. Post-Kala-Azar dermal leishmaniasis. *Int J Dermatol.,* 1995; 34: 85-91.]

Ready, P.D. and Croset, H. (1980). Diapause and laboratory breeding of *Phlebotomus* perniciosus Newstead and *Phlebotomus* ariasi Tonnair (Diptera: Psychodidae) from Southern France. *Bull. Entomol. Res., 701,* 511-23.

Regional strategic framework for elimination of *VL* from SEA Region (2005–15). New Delhi: WHO- SEARO. SEA-VBC-85 (Rev. 1), p. 22.

Regional strategic framework for elimination of *VL* from SEA Region (2005-15). New Delhi: WHO-SEARO. SEA-VBC-85 (Rev. 1), p. 22) (Communicable diseases: Kala-Azar status in SEA region 2005 (online). Available at URL http://www.searo.who.int/en/Section10/Section2163.htm.

Rehman, S.J. (1986). Reference from Manual on Entomology in *Visceral Leishmaniasis.* By Kalra N.L. and Bang Y.H. pp. 30-33.

Rioux, J.A. and Golvan, Y.J. (1963). Epidemiologie des leismanioses dans le sud de la France (English Version) Monograph 37: *(Institut National de la Sante et de la Recherche Medicale, Paris). p. 223.*

Rudin, W., Hecker, H. (1982). Functional morphology of the midgut of a sandfly as compared to other hematophagous nematocera. *Tissue Cell 14*: 751-58.

Salotra, P., Raina, A., and Ramesh, V. (1999). Western blot analysis of humoral immune response to *Leishmania donovani* antigens in patients with post Kala-Azar dermal leishmaniasis. *Transactions of Royal Society of Tropical Medicine and Hygiene., 93: 98-101.*

Salotra, P.D., Chauhan, D., Ralhan, R. and Bhatnagar, R. (1995). Tumour necrosis factor-alpha induces preferential expression of stress proteins in virulent promastigites of *Leishmania donovani. Immunology Letters, 44,* 1-5.

Sanyal, R.K., Alam, S.N., Kaul, S.M. and Wattal, B.L. (1979). Some observation on epidemiology of current outbreak of Kala-Azar in Bihar. *Journal Communicable Disease, 11:* 170.

Sanyal, R.K., Alam, S.N., Kaul, S.M. and Wattal, B.L. (1979). Some observation on epidemiology of current outbreak of Kala-Azar in Bihar. *Journal Communicable Disease, 11:* 170.

Sanyal, R.K., Banerjee, D.P., Ghose, T.K., Ghose, J.N., Mishra, B.S., Roy, Y.A., and Rao, C.K. (1979). A longitudinal review of Kala-Azar in Bihar. *J. Commun. Dis.* (1979). 11 *149.*

Schalling, H.D.F.H., Schoone, G.J., Kroon, C.C.M., Hailu, A., Chappuis, F. and Veeken, H. (2001). Development and application of 'simple' diagnostic tools for *Visceral leishmaniasis. Medical Microbiology and Immunology, 190,* 69-71.

Sen Gupta, P.C. Kala-Azar in Bengal—Its incidence and trends. *Ind. Med Gaz., 79 p. 547.*

Service, M.W. Moquito ecology- field sampling methods. Applied Science Publishers Ltd, (London).

Service, M.W., Mosquito ecology—Field sampling methods. Applied Science Publishers Ltd. (London).

Shannon, C.E. and Wiener, W. (1949). The mathematical theory of communication (Urbana, IL : University of Illinois Press).

Sharma and Dhiman (1993). Effects of Neem Extracts on *Phlebotomus* argentipes and *P. papatasi. J. Commun. Dis., 179-84.*

Sharma, M.I.D., Suri, J.C., Kalra, N.L. and Mohan, K. (1973). Habitat and Bionomics of Phlebotomine sandflies. *J. Comm. Dis. 5:* 149.

Sharma, N.L., Mahajan, V.K., Ranjan, N., Negi, A.K., Inder, K., Mehta, S., The sandflies of the Satluj river valley, Himachal Pradesh (India): Some possible vectors of the parasite causing human cutaneous and visceral leishmaniases in this endemic focus. *J Vector Borne Dis.*2009; *46:* 136-40.

Sharma, V.P. and Ansari, M.A. (1994). Personal protection from mosquitoes (Order: Diptera) by burning neem oil in kerosene. *J. Med. Entomol., 31:* 505.

Sharma, V.P., Ansari, M.A. and Razdan, R.K. (1993). Mosquito repellent action of Neem (*Azadirachta indica)* oil. *J. Ammosq Cont Assoc., 9:* 359.

Shaw, J.J. and Lainson, R. (1968). Leishmaniasis in Brazil. II. Observations on enzootic rodent leishmaniasis in the Lower Amazon Basin region – The feeding habits of the vector, Lutzomyia flaviscutellata in reference to man, rodents and other mammals. *Trans R Soc Trop Med Hyg, 62:* (1968) 396.

Shaw, J.J., Lainson, R., Ryan, L., Braga, R.R., McMahon-Pratt, D. and David, J.R. (1987). Leishmaniasis in Brazil: XXIII. The identification of *Leishmania braziliensis* in wild caught Neotropical sandflies using monoclonal antibodies. *Transactions of the Royal Society of Tropical Medicine and Hygiene, 81:* 69-72.

Singh, K.V. (1996). Susceptibility status of *Phlebotomus papatasi* and *Sergentomia punjabensis* (Diptera: Psychodidae) to some insecticides in District Bikaner (Rajasthan). *J. Commun. Dis. 28:* 28-32.

Singh, K.V. and Bansal, S.K. (1996). Insecticide susceptibility of *Phlebotomus papatasi* to organochlorine, organophosphate and carbamate compounds in some arid areas of western Rajasthan. *Indian.J. Med. Res.*, 103: 9193.

Singh, N., Mishra, A.K. and Saxena, A. (1996). Use of neem cream as a mosquito repellent in tribal areas of Central India. *Indian J. Malariol, 33:* 99, (1996.)

Singh, R., Lal, S., Saxena, V.K., Breeding ecology of visceral leishmaniasis vector sandfly in Bihar state of India. *Acta Tropica.* 2008; *107(2):* 117-20. doi: 10.1016/j.actatropica.2008.04.025) 37) (mohfw.nic.in/NRHM/Presentations/NVBDCP.pps).

Singh, S., Kumar, V. and Singh, N. (2002). Predicting Kala-Azar disease manifestation in asymptomatic patients with latent *Leishmania donovani* infection by detection of antibody against recombinant K39 antigen. *Clinical and Diagnostic Laboratory Immunology. 9,* 568-72.

Singh, S.P., Raghavendra, K., Singh, R.K. and Subbarao, S.K. (2002) Studies on larvicidal properties of leaf extract of *Solanum nigrum Linn* (Family: Solanaceae). *Curr Sci. 81:* 1529, 2002.

Sinton, J.A. (1924). Notes on some Indian species of the genus *Phlebotomus*. VIII Records of the geographical distribution and seasonal prevalence of known Indian and Cingalise species of the genus *Phlebotomus. Indian. J. Med. Res., 12: 1*035-149.

Sinton, J.A. (1925). Notes on some Indian species of the genus *Phlebotomus*. Part XII. *Phlebotomus* argentipes Annandale and Brunetti. (1908). *Indian J. Med. Res. 12:* 789-99.

State Kala-Azar data. available at URL http://nvbdcp.gov.in/iec.html – Kala-Azar/Guidelines for Vector Control in KA Elimination).

Sukumar, K., Perich, M.J. and Boobar, L.R. (1991). Botanical derivatives in mosquito control : A Review. *J. Am. Mosq. Cont. assoc. 7:* 210.

Sundar, S., Rai, M. Laboratory Diagnosis of Visceral Leishmaniasis. *Clin Diag Lab Immunol,* 2002; 9: 951-8.

Sundar, S., Reed, S.G., Singh, V.P., Kumar, P.C.K., Murrary, H.W. Rapid accurate field diagnosis of visceral leishmaniasis. *Lancet* 1998; 351: 563-5.

Sundar, S., Rosenkaimer, F., Makharia, M.K., Goyal, A.K., Mandal, A.K., Voss, A., *et al.* Trial of oral miltefosine for visceral leishmaniasis. *Lancet* 1998; 352: 1821-23.

Swaminath, C.S., Shortt, H.E. And Anderson, L.A.P. (1942). Transmission of Indian Kala-Azar to man by bites of *Phlebotomus argentipes. Indian Journal Medical Research 30,* 473-77.

Swaminath, C.S., Shortt, H.E. and Anderson, L.A.P. (1942). Transmission of Indian Kala-Azar to man by bites of *Phlebotomus argentipes*. Ann. And Brun. India. *Indian Journal of Medical Research, 30:* 473-77.

Thakur, C.P. (2001). Changing Scenario of Kala-Azar (*Visceral leishmaniasis*) in Bihar. Strategies for control of Kala-Azar and Malaria [*Proceedings of WHO Workshop] 27-28 December, 2001 organized by Balaji Utthan Sansthan Kala-Azar research centre, Patna.* PP. 1-10.

Thapar, B.R., Joshi, R.D., Rao, J.S. and Saxena, N.B.L. (1993). Status of *Phlebotomus papatasi scopoli* (Diptera: Pschycodidae) to chlorinated hydrocarbons in Panchmahal district of Gujrat state (India). *J. Commun. Dis., 25(4):* 212-13.

V. Kumar, S. Bimal, S. Keshari, A.J. Kumar, A.K. Bagchi, M.A. Akbar, K. Kishore, S.K. Bhattacharya and P. Das. (2005). Evaluation of a dot-immunoblot assay for detecting leishmanial antigen in naturally infected *Phlebotomus argentipes* (Diptera: Psychodidae). *Annals of Tropical Medicine and Parasitology, 99(4),* 371-76.

Vyokov, V.N. (1980). Control of sandflies. WHO traveling seminar on leishmaniasis control. *Moscow* (1980). PP. 11.

Wermelinger, E.D., (1990). Studies on sandfly fauna (Diptera: Psychodidae) in the focus of *Cutaneous leishmaniasis* in Mesquita, *Rio de Janeiro State, Brasil. Mem Inst Oswaldo Cruz, 85:* 39-45.

Wigglisworth, V.B., (1972). *The Principles of Insect Physiology.* 7th Edition. English language book society, Chapman and Hall. PP. 117-18.

www.msfindia.org

Yeats, D.K. (1994). The cladistics and classification of the Bombyliidae (Diptera: Asiloidea); *Bull. Am. Mus. Nat. Hist., 219:* 1-191.

Yong, T.C.M., Richmond, A.E., and Brandish, G.R. (1926). Sandflies and sandfly fever in Peshawar district. *Ind. J. Med. Res., 13:* 691-1021.

Young, TC., Mc Combie, (1924). Kala-Azar in Assam. (H.K. Lewis, London).

Zahar, A.R. (1979). Studies on leishmaniasis vectors/reservoirs and their control in the old world. WHO/VBC, *79:* 749.

Zijistra, E.E., Musa, A.M., Khalil, E.A., el-Hassan, I.M., el-Hassan A.M. PostKala-azar dermal leishmaniasis. *Lancet Infect Dis.,* 2003; 3: 87-98.

Zijlstra, E.E., Musa, A.M., Khalil, E.A.G., El Hassan, I.M., El-Hassan, A.M. Post-Kala-Azar dermal leishmaniasis. *Lancet Infectious Diseases.* 2003; 3: 87-97.

Zijltra, E.E., EL-Hassan, A.M., Ismael, A. Endemic Kala-Azar in eastern Sudan: Post-Kala-Azar dermal leishmaniasis. *Am J Trop Med Hyg.,* 1995; 52: 299–305.

□□□